Narcissistic Patients and New Therapists

Narcissistic Patients and New Therapists

Conceptualization, Treatment, and Managing Countertransference

Edited by
Steven K. Huprich

JASON ARONSON

Lanham • Boulder • New York • Toronto • Plymouth, UK

Published in the United States of America
by Jason Aronson
An imprint of Rowman & Littlefield Publishers, Inc.

A wholly owned subsidiary of
The Rowman & Littlefield Publishing Group, Inc.
4501 Forbes Boulevard, Suite 200, Lanham, Maryland 20706
www.rowmanlittlefield.com

Estover Road
Plymouth PL6 7PY
United Kingdom

British Library Cataloguing in Publication Information Available

Library of Congress Cataloging-in-Publication Data

Narcissistic patients and new therapists: conceptualization, treatment, and managing
countertransference / edited by Steven K. Huprich.
    p. ; cm.
  Includes bibliographical references and index.
  ISBN-13: 978-0-7657-0562-4 (cloth: alk. paper)
  ISBN-10: 0-7657-0562-1 (cloth: alk. paper)
  eISBN-13: 978-0-7657-0621-8
  eISBN-10: 0-7657-0621-0
  1. Narcissism—Treatment. 2. Countertransference (Psychology) I. Huprich,
Steven Ken, 1966–
  [DNLM: 1. Narcissism. 2. Countertransference (Psychology) 3. Personality
Disorders—pathology. 4. Personality Disorders—therapy. 5. Psychotherapy—
methods. WM 460.5.E3 N2222 2008]

  RC553.N36N372 2008
  616.85'854—dc22

                                                                2008030520

Printed in the United States of America

♾™ The paper used in this publication meets the minimum requirements of
American National Standard for Information Sciences—Permanence of Paper
for Printed Library Materials, ANSI/NISO Z39.48-1992.

Contents

1   Introductory Remarks   1
    Steven K. Huprich

2   Narcissistic Personality Disorder   5
    Eamonn Arble, Chelsea R. Dean, Anatol Tolchinsky,
    Steven K. Huprich

3   The Case of Mr. Garcia   23
    Courtney E. Fons

4   The Case of Mr. Miller   47
    J. Robert Parker

5   The Case of Mr. Schultz   69
    Lazslo A. Erdodi

6   The Case of Mr. Edwards   95
    Scott R. Brown

7   Closing Remarks   123
    Steven K. Huprich

Index   129

1

Introductory Remarks

Steven K. Huprich

Sometimes, good ideas come to us in surprising ways. This was certainly the case during fall semester, 2006. I was facilitating a group supervision meeting, in which my supervisees took turns throughout the semester presenting a case to the group. Our meetings lasted for one hour, which provided plenty of opportunity for discussion and reflection. Four students had been working with patients who had notable narcissistic conflicts and/or a narcissistic personality. It seemed as if this was becoming a theme of our group. And, as their supervisor, I certainly found myself experiencing a "déjà vu" with each student in the supervision process.

One day, a student was presenting, and the focus centered on his countertransference reaction to the patient. As I watched the student present the case, I found that many other students were nodding in agreement with what they were hearing. Occasionally, a smile appeared on a student's face as s/he recognized some very familiar types of experiences in the therapeutic hour. I observed how familiar this all sounded. The students readily agreed, to which I noted how much opportunity we had this semester to learn about narcissistic personalities and conflicts. Parenthetically, I stated that we were getting pretty good at recognizing these kinds of conflicts, particularly those of our own reactions to patients with these conflicts. I added that maybe we ought to write a book about this. Everyone smiled and recognized how much their experiences with these patients had helped them develop professionally. At this point, the idea seemed to take life in our group. After a brief discussion with students about whether I ought to look into this idea further, we came to an agreement that I should do just that.

The next steps happened rather fast. I made a few phone calls and was put in contact with Mr. Arthur Pompino at Rowman and Littlefield Publishers.

We discussed the idea, which was presented to the editorial staff. They liked the idea, and consequently, by April 2007, we had a contract in hand. We proceeded with our writing, and the book that you are about to read is the final product of these efforts.

As the process of writing unfolded, certain things became clear about what it was that we were creating. These could be broken down into two categories: what this book is and what it is not. I shall address the former first. This book is the product of students' learning experiences. As we all know, learning often occurs through a process of trial-and-error. We do not become good therapists without first experiencing what it means to conduct psychotherapy, to be with our patients in the room, and to reflect upon what it is that we have done well and things we have not done so well. It takes time, energy, patience, and grace to learn how to hear and be with our patients in their struggles. It also takes some work to learn how to tolerate discomfort in ourselves and our patients. As the authors will demonstrate in their chapters, they were therapists in training, striving to reach their potentials. They boldly describe their effort and show considerable courage in sharing with the reader their learning process.

Related to the above, it should be noted that this is a book from beginning therapists about their reactions to working with what are considered typically "difficult to treat" patients. The authors of the chapters were instructed to spend a considerable amount of time writing about their countertransference experiences of their patients. In doing so, the authors bear to us a part of their psyche. These experiences allow the reader to see how individualized reactions to patients actually inform treatment in two ways. First, these reactions tell something about how the patient may be experienced by others, which will be discussed in greater length in the next chapter. Second, these reactions inform the therapist about him or herself. By maintaining an openness and curiosity to what is experienced, therapists come to recognize and accept their reactions as genuine, real, and understandable. Whether the reaction is rational or irrational, the reaction or experience is now in a new sphere of understanding, which provides for greater self-understanding and a more enriched sense of self-efficacy. Subsequently, therapists learn about themselves and use this new knowledge to inform how they work with their patients.

The patients we describe herein entered into a therapy relationship and have worked very hard to better understand themselves. They have maintained an unwavering commitment to their treatment and understanding those parts of themselves that are confusing and distressing. Week after week, hour upon hour, they have done the difficult *work* of psychotherapy. All of us commend and value our patients' dedication to bettering themselves and to working within the nature of a therapeutic relationship. We are honored to be given the privilege of entering their lives and learning about their joys, hopes, conflicts, pain, and suffering. We recognize that this is "sacred" ground, and we thank patients sharing it with us. It also should be recognized that students' work with patients was supervised by many individuals. Besides myself, Drs. Norman Gordon, Karen Saules, Michael Shulman, Tamara Penix Loverich, Ellen Koch, Flora Hoodin, Carol Freedman-Doan, and Nina Nabors have provided hours of clinical supervision to the authors of these chapters. Their efforts helped the student therapists maintain the therapeutic relationship and develop their interventions accordingly.

Related to the above, the therapy experiences described herein are the product of clinical supervision and case conceptualization from multiple perspectives, within a generalist model of clinical training in an APA-approved PhD program in clinical psychology. Psychodynamic theory and attention to countertransference were not always the focus of clinical supervision and subsequent interventions. Though the authors demonstrate a psychodynamic way of thinking and conceptualizing their cases, it will be clear that their interventions reflect the breadth of models to which they were exposed.

These are partial representations of what this book is. No doubt, readers will have their own opinions of what this book has to offer and what they value about it. But for all that the book is, it is necessary to highlight what this book is not, so that one's expectations and a priori ideas can be kept in check. First of all, this book is not a detailed description of session-by-session accounts of psychotherapy, nor does it offer a verbatim account of what transpired in the clinical sessions. Cases are presented in summary format, and major themes or portions of themes within a session are described with the attempt to capture many of the trends observed in working with patients in psychotherapy.

Second, this book is not a primer of psychodynamic therapy for narcissistic patients. Because students' training is broad, and because their exposure to psychoanalytic and psychodynamic ideas is only part of their education, the treatment described in this text is not fully representative of the psychodynamic paradigm. Though supervision with me was analytically and dynamically focused, and interventions that were implemented reflected these models, the reader may be disappointed if s/he is hoping for extensive descriptions of what psychodynamic therapy looks like.[1] Nevertheless, cases are conceptualized and written from a psychoanalytic and psychodynamic perspective.

In sum, it is my hope that readers of this book will appreciate it for what it is—an honest attempt to describe and understand a patient and the therapist's reaction to the patient. Because all of the patients have narcissistic pathology of some kind, there is a natural focus in treatment on how the patient's sense of self is developed and maintained. Not surprisingly, this kind of work was also very useful for the treating clinician. It can be quite therapeutically beneficial to work with patients whose sense of self is troubled by also focusing considerable attention upon one's own sense of self, especially in the context of working with this particular patient. With this being said, let us move onto an understanding of narcissistic personality dynamics and relevant issues in conceptualization and treatment.

NOTE

1. On a personal note, it is disappointing that students are not exposed to more psychoanalytic and psychodynamic theory as part of their training. Generalist models of training do not allow the kind of depth that would provide more optimal training in psychoanalytic and psychodynamic psychotherapy. Nevertheless, in an era when these models are in decline, I am appreciative that I can still teach students these things and that they can be exposed to local training opportunities at the nearby Michigan Psychoanalytic Institute. Fortunately, greater recognition for psychoanalytic and psychodynamic approaches is being obtained. The interested reader is directed to Nancy McWilliams' books, *Psychoanalytic Diagnosis* (1994), *Psychoanalytic Assessment* (1999), *Psychoanalytic Psychotherapy* (2004)—all published by Guilford Press—or to my recent text, *Conceptual and Empirical Foundations of Psychodynamic Therapy* (2008), published by Taylor and Francis Publishers.

2

Narcissistic Personality Disorder

Eamonn Arble, Chelsea R. Dean, Anatol Tolchinsky,
Steven K. Huprich

BRIEF HISTORY

In *Metamorphoses*, Ovid tells the story of a Nymph named Echo who could only speak by repeating the phrases uttered by others. This curse was bestowed upon her by the goddess, Hera, a punishment for distracting her and allowing Zeus to successfully hide his infidelities. Echo one day fell in love with Narcissus, an arrogant young man whose beauty was said to rival that of Apollo. When Narcissus entered into her woods, she followed him, eager to cry out, but unable to do so. Eventually, upon realizing that he had become separated from his companions, Narcissus cried out, "Is anyone here?" Echo joyfully replied "Here," and rushed to embrace him. Scornfully, Narcissus rejected her, just as he had done with countless other potential lovers. Echo became so overcome with grief that she faded away until nothing but her voice remained. The goddess, Nemesis, angered by Narcissus's shallow and uncaring nature, doomed him to fall in love with his own reflection. As foretold, Narcissus would one day peer into Echo's pond, see his reflection, and fall madly in love with himself. He would retain that loving gaze upon his own image until he died.

The character of Narcissus was first used by Ellis (1898) to describe an observed disorder known at the time as male autoeroticism. This name was initially used to describe a specific kind of sexual dysfunction in which men were attracted, and sometimes even infatuated, with themselves. Freud would later apply the term "narcissistic" in *Three Essays on the Theory of Sexuality* (Freud, 1905). Freud was intrigued by this phenomenon and began to consider how it applied to patients within his developing psychoanalytic framework. In 1914 he published one of his most celebrated works: *On*

Narcissism. This seminal effort would form the foundation for all subsequent psychodynamic investigations into the narcissistic personality disorder (Chessick, 1985).

Though it is beyond the scope of this chapter to fully address Freud's conceptualization, reference to his noted U-tube analogy may prove helpful. According to Freud, narcissism was a state in which an individual's libidinal energy was directed toward the self (as opposed to outside objects). In Freud's view, in the initial phase of life, an individual's entire libido is stored within the ego, a state described as primary narcissism (a normal aspect of development). In the child's second year, s/he passes beyond the autoeroticism of primary narcissism, and develops the ability to direct those energies outward (flowing through the tube). Such a flow of libidinal energy away from the self and toward external objects granted the child the capacity for object love—love of objects other than the self. However, these libidinal energies were assumed to flow back and forth, i.e. moving between the self and outside objects. In the face of various traumas, the libidinal energy could be withdrawn back into the ego, and these instances were to be described as secondary narcissism. Thus, the reemergence of narcissism in later stages of life (i.e. secondary narcissism) was thought to be pathological, while the initial concentration of libido in the ego (i.e. primary narcissism) was not.

Although *On Narcissism* was undoubtedly influential, some of the content was largely controversial and unclear. Reich (1960), building upon Freud's work, solidified a model of narcissism compatible with the classical drive theory. As Freud had suggested, she argued that narcissism is best understood as a pathological investment of libido in the self, thereby preventing the development of object love. Unfortunately, such a view did not give cause for optimism when attempting to treat the narcissistic patient. Both Freud and Reich believed that the development of secondary narcissism prevented patients from establishing an object-related transference (Chessick, 1985). Thus, the effectiveness of psychoanalytic interventions was believed to be highly limited.

Given this highly pessimistic climate surrounding the disorder, the developments to be discussed are rendered all the more extraordinary. The transition of narcissism from a vague and possibly untreatable disorder to the highly complex and energetically explored pathology of today is remarkable indeed. What follows is an assessment of the etiology, presentation, and treatment of the narcissistic character, each addressed in turn.

THEORIES OF NARCISSISM

The two most influential theorists in the narcissistic personality disorder (NPD) literature are Otto Kernberg (1967, 1970, 1974a, 1974b, 1998) and Heinz Kohut (1971, 1977, 1984). The work of these two researchers has dominated the field of narcissistic research for several decades and remains crucial in contemporary discussions. Kohut and Kernberg offer significantly different discussions of the narcissistic personality in terms of psychoanalytic understanding, treatment approaches, and its development across the lifespan.

Kernberg (1967, 1970, 1974a, b, 1998) describes the narcissist as an arrogant, aggressive, and overtly grandiose individual. This description is the product of Kernberg's belief that the narcissistic individual's defensive organization is highly similar to that of the borderline personality disorder. Indeed, it was Kernberg's contention that the narcissistic individual operates at a borderline level of character organization. What distinguished the narcissistic individual was his/her grandiose, but nonetheless integrated, sense of self. Although they repeatedly employ primitive defenses that are characteristic of borderline levels of organization (e.g., splitting, devaluing), they tend to have a consistent and relatively functional self-structure. For the narcissistic individual, the ideal self, the ideal object, and the real self have been joined into one entity. The narcissist identifies with his/her idealized self-image in the hope of severing any dependency on other people (external objects) as well as the inner images of those objects (Gabbard, 1983). Furthermore, narcissistic individuals deny the existence of personality traits that would conflict with their idealized self-image by projecting them onto others. Consequently, others are often devalued because they come to represent the very traits that the narcissist must combat. Accordingly, narcissistic individuals are often described as exploitive and self-absorbed.

Kernberg argued that narcissistic grandiosity is a pathological process in development. Its origin is found within the narcissistic patient's difficult childhood. It is asserted that the child is confronted with cold and antagonistic parents. The parents' behavior toward the child alternates between a frigid indifference and an undercurrent of aggression and resentment. Nonetheless, the child is typically assigned a special role within the family dynamic (e.g., s/he has special talents, such as being the "smart one" in the family). The child attempts to use this special position as a way to protect himself/herself against the parents' negativity, yet such a strategy is ultimately pathological, as the parents do not always acknowledge the child's special nature. After repeatedly enduring the onslaught of the parents, the child is left with nothing but an internalized sense of specialness to return to. To escape the reality of the rejecting parents, the child learns to regard its "special position" as a way to split away from reality (i.e. the uncaring parents). Rather than integrating positive and negative representations of the self, the child only internalizes the positive and idealized facets of himself/herself and of the external objects that are confronted. The child simultaneously "splits" himself/herself (dissociates) from the negative characteristics of the self and projects them onto others.

A strongly contrasting theory may be found in the works of Heinz Kohut. Kohut's self psychology (1971, 1977, 1984), and subsequent view of narcissism, is often described as a reflection of his work with the outpatient populations he was treating (Gabbard, 1989). Although Kohut did not deny the existence of the narcissistic personality as it was currently understood, he noted that a number of his clients did not seem to fit within the standard theoretical framework. Rather, these patients tended to complain of a nondescript malaise in their lives, a sense of dissatisfaction with themselves and their relationships. They were plagued by a highly fragile self-esteem that would experience great injury if they sensed a hint of derision or disapproval from those around them.

To resolve this confusion, Kohut began to devise an alternate understanding of the narcissistic pathology. Interestingly, according to Kohut's formulation, narcissism is actually a normal developmental process. Healthy self-esteem and pathological grandiosity exist on the same continuum. The presence or absence of grandiosity is not what identifies one as narcissistic, but rather, its internalization is what separates the healthy individual from the narcissistic counterpart.

Kohut argued that as early as childhood, individuals have a "grandiose self," which represents their normal development of ambitions for power and admiration. If parents fail to meet the child's need for admiration (termed "mirroring"), the child's sense of self begins to diminish and s/he behaves in a grandiose manner in an unconscious bid to earn the parents' admiration. Similarly, children have a need to idealize their parent. However, if the parent fails to provide a model worthy/accepting of admiration, the child's sense of self is equally disturbed. Essentially, in the absence of either of these elements, the child's development becomes frozen until these needs can be fulfilled (Kohut derived much of this understanding from his analysis of these patients' therapeutic transference, the bulk of which will be explored later).

Though the two theories offer obviously differing etiological processes, Kernberg and Kohut's ideas about narcissism also may be compared via their understanding of object relatedness (or object-relations) within their patients. Object-relations refer to the self-structure internalized in early childhood which guides the formation and continuance of future relationships. More broadly defined, object-relations are the "mental representations one has of oneself and others, which appear to originate early in development, and play a substantial role in how one thinks, feels, and acts toward self and others" (Huprich & Greenberg, 2003, p. 666). These early-formed representations have a powerful effect upon an individual's interpersonal relationships. Historically speaking, narcissistic pathology was described as a form of maladaptive object-relations. Freud (1914) suggested that narcissism resulted from the transfer of the libido from the object to the ego. In the most adaptive developmental process, one would pass through a stage of primary narcissism and progress to object love. Thus, narcissism was something to be outgrown (though everyone was believed to have at least some element of narcissism within them) as primary narcissistic strivings had to be pushed aside. In other words, the two may be considered as having a negatively correlated relationship (as one's narcissism diminished, their capacity for object love increased). Like Freud, Kernberg (1970, 1974a, b, 1998) believed that narcissistic patients needed to overcome their excessive self-love in order to develop their capacity for object love.

Kohut's position was significantly different (1971). He argued that to understand object-relations one must understand narcissistic strivings and how they are met and internalized. The weight of Kohut's argument lies on his distinction between object love and object-relations (Son, 2006). He refers to the concept of a selfobject. A selfobject is another person (an object) who is perceived as part of the self (much as the child will initially view the mother as a part of himself/herself). In Kohut's understanding, before a sense of self can be developed, interactions with others must take place (indeed, the character of these interactions will be immensely important). Positive interactions with selfobjects will lead to a more mature form of narcissism and the development of the self (the process of transmuting internalization). According to Kohut, individuals always require the validation of selfobjects. However, the failure to navigate this developmental process will lead the individual continually to view objects as part of the self in an immature and inappropriate fashion. Thus, although all individuals occasionally view others as selfobjects, narcissistic individuals are not engaging in mutually loving relationships because their excessive perception of others as selfobjects prevents them from fully appreciating the distinct and separate existence that these objects enjoy. Object love requires the kind of "separation of self and object" that the narcissistic individual has not developed. Kohut concludes that narcissism is not a lack of object-relations, but merely a form of object-relations where the objects are pathologically seen as part of the self.

NORMATIVE VS. PATHOLOGICAL NARCISSISM

Though narcissistic persons were first conceptualized as psychotic individuals who represented a subtype of schizophrenia (Akhtar, 1981), Reich (1960) explored the notion that people with this sort of pathology should not necessarily be classified so harshly. The grandiose sense of self at the heart of this disorder was not found to be entirely unique. In some fashion, clients across a spectrum ranging from severely disordered to highly functional appeared to have an element of grandiosity within them. Furthermore, this sense of grandiosity, when harnessed and expressed properly, had certain adaptive qualities. The more accurate assessment, it seemed, was to note that narcissistic elements were largely ubiquitous, and appeared to operate on a continuum ranging from the normative to the pathological.

It requires little consideration to identify the potentially beneficial elements within narcissism. The artist who boldly commits to his vision and refuses to acknowledge the criticisms given by reviewers, the business-woman whose unshakeable faith in her plans inspires confidence in her bosses and subordinates alike, or the professional athlete who seemingly lives for the roar of the crowd—any of these individuals could prove to be narcissistic. And yet, it is equally plausible to suggest that these individuals are quite healthy and could be celebrated for their strength of personality. How then does one differentiate between adaptive grandiosity (or mild arrogance) and the pathological vanity found within the narcissistic personality disorder?

In a therapeutic sense, this dilemma may be resolved by assessing the quality of the individual's interpersonal relationships. Those with the more adaptive forms of narcissism display a sense of concern regarding other people's feelings, and have a genuine interest in the lives and ideas of people that are close to them. They are able to maintain long-term relationships without demanding particular benefits, because the relationship is seen as an end in itself. Furthermore, they work to resolve conflicts within the relationship, understanding their own contributions to the problems and solutions that are encountered.

This stands in stark contrast to the coldly devaluing nature of the narcissistic personality disorder. One of the fundamental features of this pathology is the self-gratifying use of friends and acquaintances. These individuals demonstrate an intense preoccupation with their personal desires and feelings, largely at the expense of those around them (Westen, 1990). Other people are not considered to have their own unique existence, needs, or feelings. Rather, they are viewed as objects to be used and taken advantage of. Typically, the breaking point of such relationships occurs when demands are made on the relationship that do not coincide with the narcissistic person's needs or expectations. Whereas a normally functioning individual would typically attempt to compromise with the person involved in their life, the narcissist will likely respond with hostile devaluating and rejection.

CLINICAL PRESENTATION

The clinical presentations of the narcissistic personality disorder are highly diverse. Because their grandiosity and inordinate self-focus are rationalized as being justified, narcissistic patients often enter therapy due to alternate concerns—depression, relationship difficulties, or perhaps feelings of emptiness or inferiority. Despite their apparent arrogance and outward dismissal of others, the personality organization of a narcissistic individual is such that their identity and self-esteem are heavily dependent upon outside verification. Indeed, much of the narcissistic pathology represents a defense against the potentially harmful judgments that others might offer. Narcissistic personalities present with an interesting dichotomy: Though they crave the approval of others for their own sense of well being, their lack of empathy prevents them from appreciating others in a sincere way. This tenuous balance leads to hidden feelings of fragility, emptiness, and weakness (McWilliams, 1994).

The grandiosity of narcissistic individuals is manifested in their arrogance, lack of empathy, and feelings of superiority. In interpersonal relationships, others are often reduced to contrivances, mere tools used to affirm or fulfill the narcissistic individual's sense of self. They may be exploited for the narcissist's gain, and the narcissistic individual may be incapable of appreciating any grievances his/her behavior elicits. This failure to appreciate others is often present in their professional endeavors as well, as they often report feeling bored and dissatisfied. Because the narcissistic individual is driven to meet unreasonable standards of achievement by an unconscious desire to obtain external affirmation, their work is bereft of passion, interest, or intrinsic motivation (Wink, 1996).

The previously described characteristics of the narcissist are clearly represented in the DSM-IV's criteria for NPD. The DSM-IV defines NPD as "a pervasive pattern of grandiosity (in fantasy or behavior), need for admiration, and lack of empathy, beginning by early adulthood and present in a variety of contexts" (p. 717, APA, 2000). See Table 2.1 for specific DSM-IV diagnostic criteria).

The DSM-IV Text Revision (APA, 2000) reports that the prevalence of NPD ranges from 2–16% of clinical populations, and less than 1% in the general population. Further, it asserts that 50–75% of those diagnosed as NPD are male. However, recent research has suggested that the DSM may have underestimated female prevalence rates. Klonsky, Jane, Turkheimer, and Oltmanns (2002) observed narcissistic qualities among college students and found that participants who adhered to gender specific behaviors were more likely to report narcissistic qualities. Specifically, masculinity in men correlated with both self ($r = .17, p \leq .01$) and peer ($r = .25, p \leq .01$) reports of narcissism. Similarly, in women femininity correlated with both self ($r = .13, p \leq .01$) and peer ($r = .30, p \leq .01$) reports of narcissism. This suggests a relatively equal prevalence of narcissism by gender, with females exhibiting such qualities differently than males.

Some researchers have suggested that a mistaken emphasis on the masculine presentation of the narcissistic pathology has led to a failure to recognize the disorder in female patients. For example, Reich (1953) notes that among narcissistic individuals, females are more likely than males to idealize their romantic partners. Additionally, Carroll (1987) found that narcissism in males related to a high need for power, while in females, narcissism related to a decreased need for intimacy. Research also suggests that narcissistic females are less prone to physical aggression (McCann & Biaggio, 1989) and more likely to be shy (Cheek & Melchior, 1985).

FORMS OF NARCISSISM

A terse examination of the DSM-IV criteria reveals an intense focus upon the quality of grandiosity. Indeed, six of the nine criteria make reference to its outward presentation in some fashion. However, a growing amount of literature supports the notion that narcissism can be expressed in other forms, namely, in a proneness for insecurity, sensitivity, and humiliation. As the previous exploration of the Kohut-Kernberg divergence revealed, narcissism seems to operate in a grandiose "overt" form, but also in notably self-effacing and shy "covert" form.

Wink (1991) provided evidence for the presence of these two types of narcissism by computing a principal-components analysis of six Minnesota Multiphasic Personality Inventory (MMPI) scales in a sample of 350 non-clinical adults. The investigation identified two factors: Vulnerability/Sensitivity and Grandiosity/Exhibitionistic. Wink referred to them as covert and overt, respectively, a practice that will be extended for the remainder of this chapter. Subsequent analyses revealed that both factors correlated negatively with self-control, suggesting a common tendency towards impulsivity and self-indulgence. However, the covert factor was found to correlate negatively with measures of sociability, dominance, social presence, and self-acceptance, while the overt factor correlated positively with these measures. Additionally, the overt factor demonstrated a positive correlation with measures of exhibition and aggression, while the covert factor was found to positively correlate with measures of anxiety and introversion.

Wink also examined each factor in relation to ratings from the participants' spouses. According to spousal ratings, both factors related to being bossy, dishonest, intolerant, and demanding. Nonetheless, the same distinctions arose. Spousal ratings confirm the previously described characteristics of each factor, indicating that participants scoring high on the covert factor were more likely to be worrisome, emotional, defensive, and tense. In contrast, those scoring high on the overt factor were described as aggressive, outspoken, egotistical, and self-centered. The contrasting patterns of correlations strongly suggested that the narcissistic disorder is far from a monolithic construct.

In a manner similar to Wink, Gabbard (2000) describes the overt narcissist as an arrogant and demanding individual, one with an apparent need for being the center of attention. These individuals appear to act with no apparent awareness or concern for how their actions are affecting those around them. Conversationally, their dialogues tend to be thoroughly self-promoting, constituting little more than boasting about their accomplishments and attributes. Indeed, they express little interest in conversations that are not focused on their own concerns. This need to be the center of attention, and the dismissal of the desires of others, seems to prevent the possibility of a truly reciprocal exchange. Given this interpersonal selfishness and their fundamental lack of empathy, those around them may report feeling estranged or alienated.

Nonetheless, Rose (2002) found that undergraduate students meeting the criteria for overt narcissism reported high levels of self-esteem and happiness. It appears that the overt narcissist's grandiosity may represent a somewhat effective psychological defense. As described by Kernberg (1970, 1974a, b, 1988), the ideal self, the ideal object, and the real self have been joined into one entity. This merger produces the noted arrogance and selfishness. Nonetheless, the overt narcissists' unwavering belief in the idealized self grants them a kind of confidence which is often reinforced through the admiration (or the perceived admiration) of those around them.

In contrast to the overt narcissist, the covert narcissist is seen as shy, sensitive, and desperate to avoid being the center of attention. He or she is hypersensitive to the reactions of others and has a tendency to interpret criticism in every reaction. Gabbard (2000) suggests that covert narcissists' fears of being exposed and humiliated arise from a sense of shame regarding their suppressed wish to reveal their grandiose nature. "They projectively attribute their own disapproval of their grandiose fantasies onto others" (Gabbard, 1983, p. 468), and thus carefully avoid having their shameful secret revealed.

Although the intrapsychic structure is similar to that of its more obvious cousin, the covert narcissist seeks to bask in the glory of an idealized object. Because of the covert narcissist's investment in the idealized object (others), his or her grandiosity is dependent upon outside approval, and is therefore more vulnerable. This is manifested as an inhibited and cautious individual. Accordingly, covert narcissists are more likely to report feelings of unhappiness and inferiority (Masterson, 1993).

Though both forms of narcissism struggle with the maintenance of their self-esteem, the methods they adopt are notably different. Overt narcissists freely express their grandiosity in an attempt to impress those around them. That their audience may not be interested in their boasting is irrelevant; the overt narcissist successfully ignores the critique that others would offer. The covert narcissist, however, maintains his or her self-esteem by avoiding situations in which s/he would be under the scrutiny of others. Furthermore, when in the presence of others, the covert narcissist carefully considers how s/he should behave in order to avoid being embarrassed.

The contrast between the two types of narcissism in this regard merits attention. Both types wish to see themselves as individuals worthy of admiration, possessing a worth beyond that of a normal person. Yet, while overt narcissists freely express their arrogance, the covert narcissist worries that others will react negatively if they embrace their immodesty. They believe that their shameful appraisal of their fantasies is shared by others, and thus act to hide them under a veil of insecurity.

TRANSFERENCE AND COUNTERTRANSFERENCE

An historical consideration of the transference phenomena reveals an initial uncertainty as to how it should be understood (Cohen, 2002). In certain texts, Freud (1912) described transference as a form of resistance—a means through which the patient worked to avoid confronting distressing memories and feelings. However, Freud (1920) additionally spoke of transference as arising from the unconscious, a reemergence of infantile sexual impulses that were themselves resisted. Racker (1968) seized upon this incertitude and offered an enduring distinction: Transference may be seen as a method of resistance, but it may also be seen as the content which the patient is attempting to resist.[1] The clinical import of this contrast carries meaningful implications for the treatment of the narcissistic individual and will be discussed in greater detail.

Regardless of the theoretical approach taken towards the patient's transference, when undergoing such a transference, the therapist may be represented to the patient as an unsettling visage of a childhood antagonist. To mitigate the strain inherent in such a transference, a well-developed therapeutic alliance must be relied upon. In an ideal sense, the patient will utilize the therapist as a transference object, while also retaining a sufficient amount of trust in the therapist to allow him/her to provide insight and analysis. Yet, in more severely developed personality disorders, the therapeutic alliance can be markedly tenuous. In these instances, the transference may assume an alarming sense of reality, as the therapist's analytic role may be lost within the patient's fearful reaction to the transference object.

To understand the feelings elicited within the narcissistic transference specifically, a return to the description offered by Kernberg is warranted. Kernberg (1970) depicts the narcissistic individual's childhood as one filled with feelings of aggression. Although the child craves the warmth and approval of the parents, their interactions rarely contain such sentiments. Rather, the child becomes painfully aware of the parents' intrusive, disapproving, and hostile feelings. The child's view of the world becomes contaminated by these same sentiments and a pervasive sense of futility. Ultimately, the inability to procure the desired feelings of love and acceptance will give rise to feelings of rage, a defining feature of the narcissistic character. The resulting adult will fear dependency, as it is seen as form of vulnerability that will necessarily result in abuse and exploitation. Though the patient feels a need to connect with the therapist, to do so would place him or her in an unacceptable, exposed position. Such a disposition does not bode well for the creation of a therapeutic alliance.

Furthermore, disturbances in the narcissistic individual's development of object relations cause them to utilize a unique form of transference. Indeed, Freud's (1914) initial assertion was that the narcissistic character was unable to develop transference because of his/her failure to recognize the therapist as an independent object. It was not until the advancements of Kernberg (1974) and Kohut (1966) that the unique nature of narcissistic transference was recognized. Whereas most patients will project a discrete internal object onto the therapist, the narcissistic patient merely externalizes an element of their conflicted sense of themselves (McWilliams, 1994). Most typically, the therapist is seen as a representation of the negative components of the self that the patient cannot accept. Thus, the transference reactions of the patient may result in an adversarial stance being taken towards the therapist. A resulting tendency to devalue the therapist may be noted, as the patient frequently disregards the therapist's comments or insights. Furthermore, narcissistic patients often seek to control the therapist, demanding special scheduling rights or insisting upon referring to the therapist by his/her first name.

The psychic energy devoted to the denial of these transferences can be staggering (Rothstein, 1982). Under the guise of aloofness and independence, the patient presents the therapist with a derisive unwillingness to consider any attempts to analyze the transference. Kernberg (1984), among others, noted the striking inability of narcissistic patients to ponder the assessments offered by the therapist. As McWilliams (1994) argues: "Typically, their transferences are so ego syntonic as to be inaccessible to exploration; a narcissistic patient believes he or she is devaluing the therapist because the therapist is objectively second-rate" (p. 179).

These profound transference reactions often provoke an equally powerful countertransference from the therapist. The narcissistic patient's continuous devaluing of the therapist and the therapeutic process represents a tremendous difficulty for even the most seasoned analyst (Tylim, 1978). A sense of exasperation may enter into the therapy, as the therapist becomes increasingly defensive over the patient's insistence that the therapy is largely inconsequential. The assault against any positive gains made in the therapy can create a feeling of worthlessness in the therapist and may systematically erode any feelings of empathy that were initially present.

Furthermore, the enduring perception of the therapist as a selfobject (i.e. as an aspect of the patient's self, namely, the devalued portion) often contributes to the growing sense of futility that the patient's aggression has initially produced (McWilliams, 1994). This reduction of the therapist to an aspect of the patient's self represents a failure to appreciate the therapist's independence and autonomy. Accordingly, therapists may report a sense of meaninglessness, as if the patient is merely engaging in a monologue that they happen to be witness to. In response, a sense of boredom, disinterest, and irritability may result.

Additionally, the negative transferences of the narcissistic patient often provoke the therapist's own unconscious resistances. To combat the troubling feelings produced by the narcissistic patient's hostility, therapists may become insistent upon aggressively confronting the patient's defenses, regardless of the patient's readiness to do so (Cohen, 2002). This is often done under the pretense of assisting the patient, though in reality, it is frequently an unconscious effort to spare the therapist the pain of enduring the narcissist's resistances. There is a prevalent danger for the therapist to respond to the patient with reciprocal hostility, a fact exacerbated by the therapist's dwindling sense of empathy.

It should be noted, however, that contentious devaluing is not the only tenor of narcissistic transferences. An idealizing transference is also reported, though the inability to recognize it as such remains consistent. In these instances, Kernberg (1974) contends, the patient is merely projecting his or her grandiose self onto the therapist. The patient expresses a desire to emulate the therapist, often adopting his or her dress and mannerisms, asking questions about the therapist's interests in order to point out similarities, or attempting to teach the therapist about various topics through the sharing of advice, facts, and stories. Because this admiration is ultimately directed at the patient's projected sense of self, attempts to analyze the transference are often futile. As with the more negative form of transference, the ego syntonic nature of the transference renders it highly defended from an external analysis. Thus, though this positive transference may create the appearance of an engaged and trusting patient, in reality, it closely mimics the unwillingness to recognize the therapist's independence and capacity for insight seen in its more negative presentation.

In contrast to the preceding discussion, Kohut's self psychology (1971, 1977, 1984) offers a less deleterious conceptualization of the narcissistic transference. Kohut believed that narcissistic patients exhibited two kinds of transference while in session: the mirroring transference and the idealizing transference. In the former, the patient looks to the therapist for validation and approval. Kohut believed that this was an attempt to capture a missing element from childhood, namely, "the gleam in the mother's eye." Kohut argued that this need for mirroring was derived from the child's "grandiose self." This aspect of the self is the normal development of ambitious drives for power, success, and admiration. At this stage, the child is marveling in its own potential as a wonderful being and looks to have that sentiment echoed by the parent. Thus, the child sees himself/herself as "marvelous" and wants to have the parent admire him/her accordingly. When this need for mirroring is not met (i.e., the parent does not provide the necessary admiration), the child's sense of being whole is weakened. The child's self-regard is diminished, and s/he seeks to compensate for this lack of empathy by trying to "earn" the parents' admiration. The child attempts to gain perfection and begins showing off, eager to prove that s/he is worthy of the parent's love. This same pattern of seeking approval of the parent is sometimes revealed in the therapeutic relationship, as the patient tries to "earn" the therapist's admiration.

The idealizing transference, conversely, is the situation in which the therapist is perceived as an omnipotent parental figure with the power to cure all of the patient's ailments. The therapist is believed to provide a model for how to behave and what to value; indeed, the therapist is seen as an example of how to be. This relates to a second aspect of the self, the idealized parental image. Just as the child requires the admiration of the parent, he or she also seeks to return that admiration by idealizing the parent. Here, the child seeks to identify with an agent more capable than himself/herself. Although the child needs to have his/her own sense of power, s/he also looks to the parents as beings of enormous strength, a kind of idealized role model. The child begins to view the parent as an invincible figure, and this will ultimately enhance the child's sense of self. In this manner, the child identifies an idealized parental figure and becomes attached with that idealized image through the admiration of the parent. Thus, the child derives an enhanced sense of worth through his/her connection with his/her extraordinary parent. "You are a powerful being, I am part of you, and therefore, I am powerful too." Just as the failure of the parents to provide appropriate mirroring for the child can be traumatic, so, too, can a failure to provide the child with a model worthy of idealization.

In the process of normal development, the child is mirrored and is able to idealize his/her parent. However, because even the most empathic parents are unable to fully meet the child's needs for mirroring and idealization, the child is forced to establish a progressively more mature differentiation of self and object images. As the child ages, s/he realizes that the idealized parent (typically the mother) is unable to provide the perfect happiness that s/he desires (e.g. the mother might be unable to comfort the crying the child because she is occupied). Thus, the soothing function that the mother serves must be internalized in a process referred to as transmuting internalization. Essentially, the child is presented with two choices when dealing with these imperfect relationships. S/he can either internalize the missing sense of perfection within his/her own grandiose self, or s/he can develop the idealized "parent imago" where perfection is assigned to the parent. These processes allow the child to develop a cohesive sense of self through a merger of the grandiose self and the idealized parental image. In this manner, an ego structure is formed (Fenchel, 1983). The grandiose sense of self is transformed into healthy ambitions, while the idealized parent imago becomes a basis for the developing superego.

Regardless of the form of narcissistic transference encountered (mirroring or idealizing), the therapist's resulting countertransference is often best understood as a reflection of his/her own narcissistic conflicts. As previously described, the persistent reduction of the therapist to a selfobject may be an unsettling experience. Furthermore, the patient's intense sensitivity to even the most subtle of the therapist's reactions can quickly grow tiresome. Seemingly innocuous behaviors (e.g. adjusting one's position in a chair) may be taken as an indication that the therapist is bored or unhappy (Gabbard, 2000). Therapists may find themselves responding with annoyance and frustration to these concerns.

Additionally, the patient's need to identify with the therapist, and be identified with in turn, may activate unconscious conflicts within the therapist. Kohut (1971) notes that therapists often have difficulty allowing the patient to indulge in his or her idealizations, frequently regarding the idealizations as indications of insincere flattery (i.e. a form of unconscious hostility). This mistaken interpretation, combined with the uncomfortable nature of the transference, often disturb the creation of a countertransference reaction of empathy and identification (i.e. mirroring). In these instances, the therapist faces the risk of recreating a flawed parental figure who is unworthy of admiration, or that of an unnecessarily judgmental object that will not provide sufficient mirroring.

TREATMENT

In his assertion that the narcissistic pathology arises from a developmental arrest, Kohut (1972) offers a fundamental insight into how treatment should proceed. In Kohut's view, a return to the initial point of developmental arrest (i.e. when the mirroring/idealizing needs were not met) is crucial. Ideally, the therapist will evoke the patient's initial psychic structures, provide the heretofore missing elements for transmuting internalization, and allow for an alternate path of development. In this manner, the developmental arrest and resulting pathology may be undone (Alnaes, 1983). Thus, the transference is a defense to be endured in order to reach the underlying structures and narcissistic core. Kohut cautions, however, that only through significant analytic work may this outcome be achieved.

It should be noted that Kohut is not suggesting that the therapists may directly fulfill the patient's needs per se. Instead, it is the goal of the therapist to provide an empathetic sense of understanding and appreciation for the patient. Rather than aggressively confronting the transference reactions, the therapist should provide an empathetic response and use it as a means to gain an understanding of the patient's fundamental narcissistic views. Such an approach will offer two main benefits. First, the therapist may thus begin to provide the missing mirroring and idealizing components for the patient. Second, after some time has passed, the therapist may begin to offer interpretations as to how the patient views him/her, as well as how the patient relates to selfobjects (this will include the therapist as well). The patient will undoubtedly bristle at such interpretations of the transference, but this is a necessary consequence. Responding to these defenses with empathetic understanding will help to repair any damage that may have occurred to the alliance in the process. This restoration of the relationship draws notable parallels with the natural process of transmuting internalization. In both cases, the child/patient must realize that the parent/therapist cannot provide for their needs perfectly, and thus, the idealizing/mirroring functions that they perform must be internalized. The conclusion of such a therapy is that the patient is able to develop his/her previously missing psychic structures, form a cohesive sense of self (thereby developing an appropriate sense of object relations), and emerge with sensible ambitions and beliefs.

It is perhaps easiest to understand Kernberg's view of treatment through a comparison to Kohut's. Kernberg (1974) thoroughly rejects the notion of narcissism as an alternate line of development. In Kernberg's view, the narcissistic transference must be consistently and forcefully confronted (Gabbard, 2000). The narcissistic transference is viewed as a defense against the development of a mature form of object relations. Whereas Kohut believes that the narcissist is unable to acknowledge the therapist's independence (because their development has been halted), Kernberg insists that the patient refuses to do so. The narcissistic individual is supremely self-interested, and his/her defenses prompt the severe devaluing of the therapist. It is this narcissistic defense that must be undone.

Because Kernberg does not accept the notion of transmuting internalization, there is no need to retrace the progression of the patient's current psychic structures in treatment. Rather, the narcissist's reliance on the primitive defense of idealizing and devaluing is what must be addressed. The devaluing transference (i.e. the projection of the negative aspect of the self onto the therapist) must be revealed for what it is: an expression of the patient's rage and a simultaneous defense against the harm that the patient feels the therapist might inflict. Because the patient projects his/her own sadistic impulses onto the therapist, there is a constant fear of reprisal (indeed, this is displayed in other relationships as well, and contributes to the narcissist's view of the world as a hostile place). In a sense, the narcissist fully expects the therapist to be cold and rejecting in the same way the parents were, thus, devaluing the therapist is a preemptive strategy. "Who cares if the therapist disapproves, his opinion is meaningless."

Throughout the therapy, the narcissistic transferences will be regarded as a defense and will be interpreted as such. The patient must be made to recognize the immature defenses he or she is applying, and must further recognize the motivation behind the tendency to devalue. In this fashion, the narcissistic defenses may be dissolved.

As a concluding note, Kernberg (1974) was aware of the seemingly aggressive tone of his treatment approach. The narcissistic patient's tendency to devalue the therapist makes the development of empathy quite difficult, and when operating under the belief that the patient must be repeatedly challenged, the therapist's own aggressive impulses must be constantly monitored. Indeed, in certain instances, the patient may be inclined to assume that s/he is being devalued by a therapist who is forever commenting on themes of negative transference. To that end, Kernberg notes that the analyst must remain aware of the patient's capacity for love and object recognition. The fundamental principle of caring for one's patient is in no way altered in the treatment of the narcissistic pathology, it is merely more difficult to maintain.

NOTE

1. Racker (1968) argues that this distinction is responsible for the divergent treatment approaches adopted by various analysts. If transference is regarded a means of resistance, it is to be used as a way of recreating and confronting the infantile desires. Conversely, if the transference itself is the material being resisted, the infantile desires are to be used to bring the transference to consciousness.

REFERENCES

Akhtar, S., & Thomson, J. A., Jr. (1982). Overview: Narcissistic personality disorder. *American Journal of Psychiatry, 139(1)*, 12–19.

Alnaes, R. (1983). Understanding and treatment of narcissistic personality disturbances: The Kernberg-Kohut divergence, *Scand. Psychoanalytic Rev.*, 6, 97–110.

American Psychiatric Association. (APA). (1994). *Diagnostic and statistical manual of mental disorders* (4th ed.; DSM-IV). Washington DC: Author.

American Psychiatric Association. (APA). (2000). *Diagnostic and statistical manual of mental disorders*. (4th ed., rev.) Washington, DC: Author.

Carroll, L. (1987). A study of narcissism affiliation, intimacy, and power motivates among students in business administration. *Psychological Reports, 61*, 355–58.

Cheek, J. M., & Melchior, L. A. (1985). *Are shy people narcissistic?* Paper presented at the 93rd Annual Convention of the American Psychological Association, Los Angeles.

Chessick, R. (1985). *Psychology of the Self and the Treatment of Narcissism*. Northvale, New Jersey: Jason Arson.

Cohen, D. (2002). Transference and countertransference states in the analysis of pathological narcissism. *Psychoanalytic Review, 89(5)*, 631–51

Eagle, M. N. (2000). A critical evaluation of current conceptions of transference and countertransference. *Psychoanalytic Psychology, 17*, 24–37.

Ellis, H. (1898). Auto-erotism: A psychological study. *Alienist and Neurologist. 19*, 260–99.

Fenchel, G. (1983). Interaction between narcissism and masochism in the borderline personality. *Issues in Ego Psychology, 6*, 62–68.

Freud, S. (1905). *Three Essays on the Theory of Sexuality*, trans. James Strachey. New York: Basic Books.

Freud, S. (1912). The dynamics of transference. *Standard Edition, 12*, 97–108

Freud, S. (1914). On narcissism: An introduction. *Standard Edition, 14*, 67–102.

Freud, S. (1920). Beyond the pleasure principle. *Standard Edition, 18*, 1–64.

Gabbard, G. O. (2000). *Psychodynamic psychiatry*, (3rd ed.). Washington, DC: American Psychiatric Press.

Gabbard, G. (1983). Further contributions to the understanding of stage fright: narcissistic issues. *Journal of American Psychoanalytic Association, 31*, 423–41.

Gabbard, G. (1989). Two subtypes of narcissistic personality disorder. *Bulletin of the Menninger Clinic, 53*, 527–32.

Hotchkiss, S. (2005). Key concepts in the theory and treatment of narcissistic phenomena. *Clinical Social Work Journal, 33*, 127–44.

Huprich, S. K., & Greenberg, R. P. (2003). Advances in the assessment of object relations in the 1990s. *Clinical Psychology Review, 23*, 665–98.

Kernberg, O. F. (1967) Borderline personality organization. *Journal of American Psychoanalytic Association, 15*, 641–85.

Kernberg, O. (1970). Factors in the psychoanalytic treatment of narcissistic personalities. *Journal of the American Psychoanalytic Association, 18*, 51–85.

Kernberg, O. (1974a). Contrasting viewpoints regarding the nature and psychoanalytic treatment of narcissistic personalities; a preliminary communication. *Journal of the American Psychoanalytic Association, 22*, 255–67.

Kernberg, O. (1974b). Further contributions to the treatment of narcissistic personalities. *International Journal of Psychoanalysis, 55*, 215–40.

Kernberg, O. F. (1984). *Severe personality disorders: Psychotherapeutic strategies.* New Haven, CT and London: Yale University Press.

Kernberg, O. (1998). *Disorders of narcissism: Diagnostic, clinical, and empirical implications.* Washington, DC: American Psychiatric Press.

Klonsky, E. D., Jane, J. S., Turkheimer, E., Oltmanns, T. F. (2002). Gender role and personality disorders. *Journal of Personality Disorders, 16*, 464–76.

Kohut, H. (1966). Forms and transformations of narcissism. *Journal of the American Psychoanalytic Association, 14*, 243–72.

Kohut, H. (1971). *The analysis of the self.* New York: International Universities Press.

Kohut, H. (1972). Thoughts on narcissism and narcissistic rage. *Psychoanalytic Study Child, 27*, 360–400.

Kohut, H. (1977). *The restoration of the self.* New York: International University Press.

Kohut, H. (1984). *How does analysis cure?* Chicago: University of Chicago Press.

Kohut, H. (1968). The psychoanalytic treatment of narcissistic personality disorders. *Psychoanalytic Study of Children, 23*, 86–113.

Masterson, J. (1993). *The Emerging Self: A Developmental, Self, and Object Relations Approach to the Treatment of the Closet Narcissistic Disorders of the Self.* New York: Bruner/Mazel.

McCann, J. T., & Biaggio, M. K. (1989). Narcissistic personality and self-reported anger. *Psychological Reports, 64*, 55–58.

McWilliams, N. (1994). *Psychoanalytic diagnosis.* New York: Guilford.

Racker, H. (1968). *Transference and Countertransference.* New York: Int. Univ. Press.

Reich, A. (1953). Narcissistic object choice in women. *Journal of the American Psychoanalytic Association, 1*, 22–44.

Reich, A. (1960). Pathological forms of self-esteem regulation. *Psychoanalytic Study of Children, 15*, 215–32.

Rose, P. (2002). The happy and unhappy faces of narcissism. *Personality and Individual Differences, 33*, 379–91.

Rothstein, A. (1982) The implications of early psychopathology for the analyzability of narcissistic personality disorders. *Internat. J. Psycho-Anal., 63*, 177–87.

Rovik, J. (2001). Overt and covert narcissism: Turning points and mutative elements in two psychotherapies. *British Journal of Psychotherapy, 17(4)*, 435–47.

Schultz, R. E. & Glickauf-Hughes, C. (1995). Countertransference in the treatment of pathological narcissism. *Psychotherapy, 32,* 601–07.

Son, A. (2006). Relationality in Kohut's psychology of the self. *Pastoral Psychology, 55,* 81–92.

Tylim, I. (1978). Narcissistic transference and countertransference in adolescent treatment. *Psychoanalytic Study of the Child, 33,* 279–92.

Westen, D. (1990). The relations among narcissism, egocentrism, self-concept, and self-esteem: Experimental, clinical, and theoretical considerations. *Psychoanalysis and Contemporary Thought, 13,* 183–239.

Wink, P. (1991). Two faces of narcissism. *Journal of Personality and Social Psychology, 61(4),* 590–97.

Wink, P. (1996). Narcissism. In C. G. Costello (Ed.), *Personality characteristics of the personality disordered* (pp. 146–72). New York: Guilford.

Table 2.1.   DSM-IV diagnostic criteria for narcissistic personality disorder

A pervasive pattern of grandiosity (in fantasy or behavior), need for admiration, and lack of empathy, beginning by early adulthood and present in a variety of contexts, as indicated by five (or more) of the following:

(1) Has a grandiose sense of self-importance (e.g., exaggerates achievements and talents, expects to be recognized as superior without commensurate achievements)

(2) Is preoccupied with fantasies of unlimited success, power, brilliance, beauty, or ideal love

(3) Believes that he or she is "special" and unique and can only be understood by, or should associate with, other special or high status people (or institutions)

(4) Requires excessive admiration

(5) Has a sense of entitlement, i.e., unreasonable expectations of especially favorable treatment or automatic compliance with his or her expectations

(6) Is interpersonally exploitative, i.e., takes advantage of others to achieve his or her own ends

(7) Lacks empathy: is unwilling to recognize or identify with the feelings and needs of others

(8) Is often envious of others or believes that others are envious of him or her

(9) Shows arrogant, haughty behaviors or attitudes

From the American Psychiatric Association. (APA). (1994). Diagnostic and Statistical Manual of Mental Disorder (4th ed.; DSM-IV). Washington DC: Author, p 717.

3

The Case of Mr. Garcia

Courtney E. Fons[1]

CASE DESCRIPTION

Mr. Garcia was a sixty-one-year-old, Hispanic male. He was born to immigrant parents and was an only child. When Mr. Garcia originally presented for treatment, his presenting problem was severe depressive symptoms, with high levels of irritability. He came across as extremely hopeless and reported active suicidal ideation. At the time of originally seeking treatment, he had been experiencing unremitting depressive symptoms for approximately one year. He also reported experiencing conflicts in his family relationships, a lack of interpersonal relationships, and long-term distress regarding his sexual orientation.

Mr. Garcia was transferred to me by a male therapist who had seen him for approximately one year at a training clinic of a neighboring university. His treatment at this clinic was largely cognitive-behavioral in nature. According to his therapist's reports, Mr. Garcia made very minimal progress in treatment and was largely noncompliant with assignments both in and outside of sessions. This course of treatment mainly focused on Mr. Garcia's conflicts with his son, as well as his past negative professional experiences. Childhood experiences and parental relationships, as well as Mr. Garcia's sexual orientation conflict went, for the most part, unexplored. His previous therapist also reported having initial difficulty building rapport with Mr. Garcia. Specifically, he stated that Mr. Garcia initially appeared highly defensive and expressed worry regarding how the therapist would react to him. He also reported that Mr. Garcia reacted in a volatile way when informed that he would need to be referred to a new therapist. He accused his clinician of acting unprofessionally by withholding this information from him. As a result, he also failed to attend the last session, likely to avoid the pain of feeling as if he were being abandoned by his therapist.

Mr. Garcia was previously employed for twenty years as the chief executive officer (CEO) of a major manufacturing corporation. However, due to negative interpersonal relationships and poor management of stressful situations associated with his job, he was forced to retire at the age of fifty-eight. Mr. Garcia had been divorced for ten years when I began seeing him. He had full custody of a sixteen-year-old son, who was developmentally disabled and quite defiant. His son regularly abused marijuana and was frequently truant at school. Mr. Garcia's relationship with his son was highly conflictual and often verbally explosive. Despite always having a rather distant relationship with him, Mr. Garcia requested full custody because he did not trust his ex-wife to raise him properly. He also reported that he believed his relationship with his son would improve once his son became more mature and realized what a good father he had.

Although he was previously married for twelve years, Mr. Garcia identified himself as bisexual. He had had sexual contact with both men and women, but never had a serious romantic relationship with a man. He was quite conflicted about his sexual orientation as he viewed being attracted to members of the same sex as sinful. This was largely related to Mr. Garcia's devoutly Catholic religious beliefs. In his romantic life, Mr. Garcia had a history of repeatedly prematurely ending romantic relationships with women out of fear that they would hurt him. In his view, he was unable to trust his female partners since they would likely cheat on him and hurt him in some way. He held strong to this belief despite never having had a woman act unfaithfully toward him. While Mr. Garcia did not have this same fear in his relationships with men, he never felt a desire to have a long-term romantic relationship. Instead, he preferred to limit his relations with males to anonymous sexual encounters.

Mr. Garcia described his ex-wife as very passive, uneducated, and unattractive. He stated that his relationship with her was more similar to a friendship than a marriage. In fact, the two were only sexually intimate when attempting to have their son. When asked why he chose to marry her, he stated that he did not believe she would cheat on him. Though not attracted to her, he felt as though she was very much in love with him. Toward the end of their relationship, he began to feel that she no longer loved him as much as she used to. Because he feared that his wife would pursue an affair or end the relationship, he suggested that they divorce. When asked what made him believe that her love for him was lessening, he stated that she did not display the same level of concern and attention toward him as he thought he deserved.

Mr. Garcia suffered from a number of medical conditions, such as restless leg syndrome and diabetic nephropathy. While these conditions were of moderate severity, he had a tendency to describe them in a very detailed and overly dramatic manner. He also expressed a strong dislike and disapproval toward physicians, as he believed that they did not provide him with the concern and attention he deserved. This was also the case for psychiatrists from which he sought care. For example, while I was treating him, he changed psychiatrists five times in an effort to find one that would spend more than twenty minutes with him at each appointment. Even when explained that it was fairly routine for physicians only to spend this amount of time with their patients, he believed that medical professionals should recognize that his conditions were severe and that he was not a "routine" patient.

Mr. Garcia's previous therapist had diagnosed him with recurrent and severe major depressive disorder. While I agreed with this diagnosis, I began to observe strong narcissistic qualities as early as the first session. He expressed some grandiosity regarding his past professional accomplishments. For example, he seemed to selectively share those details of his professional experiences that demonstrated his uniqueness or talents, while failing to share details about any mistakes he made or problems that he encountered (which he acknowledged in the first session). Further, it appeared that he only experienced a sense of satisfaction when his talents were admired and envied by others. It seemed as if his identity and self-esteem were founded in others' affirmations of his professional talents.

Mr. Garcia placed great focus on his past career experiences, which seemed to distance him from his current life situation. Session after session, he would share very detailed and inflated stories of his career achievements. For example, he would often explicitly discuss his salary and the uniqueness of his talents relative to other business executives. In addition, he would place great focus on situations in which he was needed by others. He expressed an expectation to still be recognized by others as superior and highly talented despite being retired. There was a sense of being entitled to constant admiration from others.

Despite Mr. Garcia's demonstration of grandiosity and inflated self-esteem, he was highly sensitive to criticism and rejection from others. As was demonstrated in his behavior pattern in his relationships with women, he was highly mistrustful and strongly feared being abandoned. His deep insecurities were further demonstrated in his constant need for attention and concern from others. He was highly demanding of the people in his life and had an expectation that he would be treated like the unique and superior person he tried to project.

Mr. Garcia also seemed to lack the ability to outwardly relate to others' difficulties. This was especially exemplified in his relationship with his son, who was mildly mentally retarded and experienced symptoms of social phobia. Because of these psychological disabilities, his son had academic difficulties and rarely interacted with his peers. Mr. Garcia frequently criticized his son for his lack of academic success and seemed unwilling to recognize that his son's learning problems were largely out of his son's immediate, conscious control. He also refused to attribute his son's social deficiencies to anxiety and, instead, expressed the opinion that his son was simply unwilling or unable to make friends.

BACKGROUND

Mr. Garcia was raised on the West coast, where his parents still reside. His parents were raised in extreme poverty, in a racially mixed part of a large metropolitan city. During his upbringing, Mr. Garcia's father had a modest job in a factory, while his mother did not work outside the home. While his family was by no means wealthy, Mr. Garcia always had his basic physical needs met.

Mr. Garcia's parents were very young when he was conceived, but not yet married. Throughout his life, Mr. Garcia stated that his parents were quite vocal about not having wanted any children and being regretful about his conception. Their criticism extended into other areas of his life, which Mr. Garcia experienced mainly with his mother, who "criticized me for everything." These criticisms generally focused on him not being what she believed a "good son" should be, which included not being accepted by his peers or properly engaging in religious acts. Additionally, he shared stories of long-term physical and emotional abuse at the hands of his mother. For instance, she had a history of slapping him in the face for rather minor offenses (e.g. leaving a toy on the floor, throwing a ball in the house). In her worst moments, she also repeatedly told him that he was an incompetent son and wished he were never born. While the emotional abuse from his mother was fairly constant, the physical abuse only occurred randomly when he was alone with her, such that he was largely unable to predict what behaviors would result in his mother being violent toward him. This was particularly painful for Mr. Garcia, as it left him feeling out of control and in a constant state of fear and anxiety. As an adult, he expressed a sense of strong hatred, often bordering on disgust, toward his mother for her painful and sadistic actions toward him.

Despite his reports of his mother as abusive, Mr. Garcia held a very idealistic view of his father. In session, he would often recount instances of his father's "heroic" actions, like allowing Mr. Garcia to borrow the family car or his father's tools. He did not share negative experiences about his father and denied that his father was capable of being less-than-perfect. Despite his idealized account of his relationship with his father, the actual time the two of them spent together was minimal, since his father worked long hours. Further, Mr. Garcia had difficulty providing multiple examples of when the two spent quality time together or engaged in activities that they both enjoyed. Instead, he more frequently described instances of when he was watching his father from afar and fantasizing about the relationship the two of them had. These fantasies would often focus on his father being proud and accepting of Mr. Garcia.

Mr. Garcia reports that his father never witnessed the physically abusive acts his mother committed toward him because, if his father had known about it, he would have absolutely put a stop to it. He further struggled to recount how his father acted when his mother was emotionally abusive, and he appeared to have great difficulty accepting the ambiguity surrounding his father's reactions to him being abused. Further, Mr. Garcia was largely unwilling to examine the relationship his parents had with each other and the way in which they interacted to parent him. He found it difficult to provide any examples of positive experiences he had with them together.

Mr. Garcia reported having his first sexual encounter with an older adolescent boy when he was thirteen. This occurred in his home while his mother was present and consisted mainly of the two fondling each other's genitalia. While he expressed feeling angry toward his mother for allowing him to be alone with the adolescent boy, he did not describe the experience as being traumatic for him. Instead, he reported that he found the experience to be highly pleasurable and sexually charged. While he had felt physically attracted to males before this encounter, its occurrence left him feeling more confused and conflicted about his sexual orientation.

Throughout middle school and high school, Mr. Garcia pursued romantic and sexual relationships with females. These relationships were very brief, not lasting more than two months, and were always ended by him. In college, he began to have anonymous sexual relationships with men in addition to his relationships with women. While they occurred rather frequently, they generally left Mr. Garcia feeling very ashamed and guilty. These brief sexual relationships with men and women continued until Mr. Garcia was thirty-six. It was at this time that he met the woman that would become his wife. He decided to marry her after only two months of dating. When asked why he decided to marry her, he stated that he wanted to end his long history of sexual relationships with men and women, as he felt guilty and shameful about them. Instead, he wanted to be a "good Catholic" and get married like his mother wanted him to. He reported that, while he got along well with his wife, he was always dissatisfied with her and, with the exception of the conception of their son, they never had sexual intercourse. Since his divorce ten years ago, Mr. Garcia had not had any serious romantic relationships with men or women, although there were a few brief sexual encounters with women. In the time I treated Mr. Garcia, he denied any sexual activity or pursuing a long-term relationship.

Throughout his life, Mr. Garcia had very few close, interpersonal relationships. He shared with me several experiences of being bullied by his
peers. When describing these experiences, he expressed strong feelings of
alienation and victimization. He believed his peers did not accept him because of his ethnicity, as he was raised in a primarily Caucasian community.
He also expressed a strong belief that he would have had many friends had
he lived in a more Hispanic community. These sets of problems were attributed to his mother, as she had chosen the neighborhood in which they
lived, much like the one where she was raised. As an adolescent and adult,
Mr. Garcia enjoyed interacting with others on a casual level and reported
having many acquaintances. However, he never successfully had an intimate or long-term friendship with another person. Though he desired having closer interpersonal relationships, Mr. Garcia stated that he never found
a person he believed was deserving of his friendship.

Mr. Garcia was always a high academic achiever, having earned a 4.0
grade point average in high school. When he was eighteen-years-old, he
moved to the East coast for college. He performed well in both undergraduate and graduate school, going on to earn his doctorate in business administration. When asked why he decided to pursue this much education,
he stated that he knew the degree would bring him the wealth he desired
and would guarantee him a position where he was in charge of others. He
also believed that he would be less vulnerable to the demands of others and
would be able to make more autonomous decisions.

The onset of Mr. Garcia's depressive symptoms occurred soon after he
was fired from his last CEO position. Prior to this, Mr. Garcia was working
on merging with another company. This company was based in Honduras,
and because Mr. Garcia spoke both Spanish and English, he conducted
most of the negotiations with the Spanish-speaking president of the other
company. After the contract for the merger was negotiated and enacted, Mr.
Garcia was fired from his position because the owner of the company Mr.
Garcia worked for was not happy with the negotiated contract. Since the
owner had agreed to the contract before it was signed, Mr. Garcia felt that
the only reason he was fired was because he was Hispanic and the owner
was Caucasian. More specifically, Mr. Garcia suspected that the owner felt
that he had written the contract in favor of the merger because the owner of
that company was Hispanic.

Coinciding with his firing, Mr. Garcia began to experience a number of
medical problems. He began having complications related to his diabetes
and was diagnosed with diabetic nephropathy. As a result, he had frequent
medical appointments, underwent a number of treatments, and was limited
in his functioning. Consequently, these issues evoked ideas about Mr. Garcia's mortality, which he found difficult to integrate into his sense of identity. He quickly became hopeless and began experiencing suicidal thoughts.

He feared that he would never be able to work again, which, in his view, meant that life was not worth living. When he reported these thoughts to his physician, he was encouraged to seek psychotherapy in addition to the psychotropic medication he was already receiving.

TREATMENT HISTORY

Prior to beginning treatment with Mr. Garcia, I met with his previous therapist to discuss the case.[2] This therapist informed me that, upon learning that he would be transferred, Mr. Garcia expressed a concern that a therapist would be unable to understand his unique experience. He cited his ethnicity, intelligence, and prolific knowledge about psychotherapy as reasons why a therapist must be highly talented in order to understand him and provide him with effective treatment. When informed that I was a Caucasian female, he was highly concerned about not only my *ability* to understand him, but also my *willingness* to understand him. However, once the previous therapist shared with Mr. Garcia his opinion that I was quite capable, he seemed somewhat pacified, but stated that the therapist must still prove her talent to him.

The focus of the first session was to gain a better understanding of Mr. Garcia's background and current psychological problems. However, Mr. Garcia was only interested in discussing his concerns about my clinical skills, as well as his ability to build a therapeutic alliance with me. When these concerns were explored, he related that he was apprehensive about working with a female therapist, as he had only been treated by males in the past. When asked whether my gender made him feel uncomfortable or would impair his ability to talk openly about his problems, he stated that it would not. He stated that feeling comfortable and trusting toward his therapist was not the focus of his concern; instead, he worried that being female would impair my ability to understand him and be an effective therapist. However, when he was offered the opportunity to be transferred to a male therapist, he declined.

The next session was focused on gaining a better understanding of the history of Mr. Garcia's problems and discussing what he would like to accomplish in treatment. Toward the end of this session, Mr. Garcia began critiquing my physical appearance and attire. For example, he stated that, as a therapist, I should not wear a red blouse. When this comment was explored further, he said he preferred I wear black or gray suits, as colored clothing was distracting to him. He felt colored clothing brought too much attention to me, when the sessions should solely be focused on him. In addition, as he was exiting the office, he remarked that I should not wear any make-up during our sessions. Because this comment was made when we were a public area, I did not respond to it or attempt to explore it at that time.

At the beginning of the third session, I attempted to explore the comments that Mr. Garcia had made about my appearance and attire. When asked why he wanted to share those comments with me, he immediately became defensive and stated that he was just being honest. He stated that this is just the way he is: he speaks his mind and is not going to hold back anything in therapy. I followed this up by asking again what he had hoped my response would be to his concerns. He again stated that he was just being honest. He then shifted the focus on me, believing that I was offended by his comments. When asked a third time about concerns he might have about my attire, he again placed the focus on me by stating that I was being defensive. Recognizing that this line of inquiry was unproductive, I discontinued my questioning and accepted his answers for what they were. This interaction further supported my hypothesis that Mr. Garcia had strong narcissistic traits; he demonstrated a high sensitivity to criticism, and even though this discussion was intended to further explore his concerns about me as a therapist, he immediately interpreted the questions as direct criticism toward him. To defend himself from this perceived criticism, he turned the focus on me and became very devaluing.

A few days after this session, I was informed that Mr. Garcia had spoken with the clinic director about his concerns about me as his therapist. He stated that he did not have confidence in my clinical skills and did not believe that I could or that I genuinely wanted to understand his experience. He attributed this belief to my gender and ethnicity. In response to these concerns, the clinic director made several suggestions, including that he could be transferred to another therapist. However, he declined this offer and instead decided to pursue the clinic director's suggestion to continue to try working with me for a few more sessions. In our next meeting, I made sure I communicated to him my willingness and desire to understand him through my in-session behaviors. For example, I stated that I cared about him and wanted to try to understand him. I also closely monitored my body language and nonverbal communication to ensure that I was not accidentally conveying disinterest or discomfort. Later, I recognized that my sensitivity to him at this point was related to the strong countertransference he elicited in me, in that I saw him as quite fragile and someone who needed considerable attention so that he would not be hurt by even minor kinds of behaviors or nonverbal communication. (I will discuss this issue in greater depth later in the chapter.)

This exchange seemed to reassure him and foster the development of our therapeutic relationship. Yet, while I continued to assess and understand his background and current problems in the next few sessions, Mr. Garcia continued to be critical about the treatment and my personal characteristics. He would often compare me with his past therapists. Because I felt that therapeutic alliance was still on uncertain grounds, I began to alter my therapeutic technique. I substantially decreased the number of direct questions I would ask, which he often perceived as threatening or critical, and instead began using a more empathic, rapport building approach. I conveyed a sense of interest in understanding his experiences. When he shared experiences of victimization, as he often did, I acknowledged his feelings and empathized with his experience. When he recounted the abuse inflicted by his mother, I recognized that his basic needs were not met.

This experience demonstrated to me the great importance of empathy and reflection in the treatment of patients with narcissistic personality disorder. These techniques appeared to increase Mr. Garcia's commitment to therapy. It also helped cultivate a stronger therapeutic relationship. After consistent use of mirroring and empathic validation, Mr. Garcia conveyed a greater sense of confidence in my therapeutic skills and ability to successfully treat him. Mr. Garcia also seemed to become more comfortable focusing on himself in session, rather than me, and his associations shifted toward issues surrounding those things which conflicted him most.

Subsequently, Mr. Garcia revealed strong themes of victimization, especially with regard to his past employment. He expressed feeling as if he was not respected as highly as he should have been and was not treated as well as others were, because he was Hispanic. His subsequent associations led to devaluing his workers and focusing on how his skills or intelligence made him superior to them. When thinking of being victimized, he would focus solely on others' deficiencies or aggression and resisted identifying his role in any of these experiences. In part, this resistance was a product of his belief that he was helpless in these situations, since his ethnicity could not be changed. As these issues arose, I believed they were likely a projection of the conflicts he had about his own identity.

This trend of sharing grandiose stories or experiences of victimization continued until the ninth session, which seemed to be a turning point. Mr. Garcia presented at this session as severely depressed and hopeless. He also reported frequently contemplating suicide, following a negative experience he had with his neighbor. He reported that his neighbor, who was African American, had a party and did not invite him. Mr. Garcia believed that this was because he was Hispanic. Because he could not change his ethnicity, he expressed feeling very hopeless about his future. He expressed the belief that others' would continue to victimize him and killing himself would be the only way to avoid his years of suffering because of his ethnicity. His plan was to commit suicide by jumping off a bridge located far away from his home, as this method would best ensure that his attempt would be successful.

Because he reported serious suicidal thinking, the option of being hospitalized was discussed with him. However, he was strongly opposed to this idea. He also refused the numbers for emergency psychiatric services. He stated that he was not going to agree to any of these options, since I was just providing them to avoid being held liable. I then related with Mr. Garcia that I was genuinely concerned about his well-being and did not want him to do anything to hurt himself. This discussion completely altered Mr. Garcia's demeanor. He stated that he was surprised that I actually cared about him, and he agreed not to harm himself. By being forthright and honest about my genuine concern, Mr. Garcia finally believed that he was cared about and valued. He consequently appeared to feel more secure in the therapeutic relationship, and this seemed to change his view of me from someone that may victimize him to someone whom he could trust.

After this event, we were able to assess his suicidal thinking in more detail. Mr. Garcia's suicidal thoughts seemed to be strongly tied to his identification with his father. His idea of how he would commit suicide was not one that could be carried out in a spontaneous fashion, but was one that would require time and planning. When his suicidal ideation was further explored, it became clear that he only planned to commit suicide if his father died before his mother did. His rationale was that he did not want to be left to take care of his mother without having the protection of his father. He stated that he had no choice but to take care of his mother, believing that he owed it to his father to take care of her by taking his father's place. However, this impending responsibility was very threatening. He feared that he would again suffer at the hands of his mother. Even more threatening was the pressure Mr. Garcia put on himself to meet the idealized expectations of his father. He would need to be loving and nurturing to a woman who had caused him so much pain and anguish. For Mr. Garcia, committing suicide would be the only acceptable way for him to avoid this responsibility. In fact, when asked whether he ever contemplated having his mother put into an assisted living facility rather than him becoming her caretaker, Mr. Garcia became extremely defensive. He could not entertain the idea that he would voluntarily choose not to take care of his mother. This action would be deplorable and worthy of punishment, mainly because it was in direct opposition to how his father chose to act.

Mr. Garcia's fears of about his father dying were also related to the effect that his suicide would have on his own son. When I asked about this for the first time, he was highly resistant to discussing it further. However, sensing that the idea would be too distressing to acknowledge, I asked him about the possibility that his son could be deeply hurt and experience a profound sense of loss in response to his death. While he at first resisted answering this question, he ultimately related that he would feel important and cared about if his son was impacted by his death. Immediately after saying this, however, he stated that this would not be the case, since his disappointing son did not have the capacity to be concerned about another human being. For Mr. Garcia, it was less painful to conclude that his son was not mentally capable of loving another person, than to acknowledge that his son may care about him.

Following Mr. Garcia's suicidal crisis, additional important material regarding his relationship with his son arose. In general, he began to speak more openly about his frustrations and anger toward his son, with whom he was extremely disappointed. His associations led him to compare his son's mental illnesses and behavior problems to those of his own. He described his son as being a failure and stated that there was nothing positive about him. However, it seemed here that a large part of Mr. Garcia's concern was a projection of his own sense of inadequacy onto his son. However, when I asked how his experience of his son may be related to how he felt about himself, he stated it was not at all related. He stated that his son's anxiety and inabilities were so much more severe than his own that the two of them could not even be compared. Mr. Garcia could not even accept the suggestion that perhaps having his own difficulties could help him empathize with his son, and that he would never be able even imagine what it would feel like to be that "screwed up."

It was not surprising, then, that Mr. Garcia began to describe explosive outbursts he had when his son did not fulfill his expectations of how a son should treat his father, even though these expectations were lofty and, at times, unrealistic. For example, he shared an instance in which he had decided to go to the movies. When he asked his son if he would like to go with him, his son stated that he was tired and wanted to go to bed early instead. Mr. Garcia reacted to this response with extreme anger and frustration. As we explored his anger, Mr. Garcia defended his expectations that his son should have wanted to go with him. He also compared his son's behavior to how he would have reacted if his father had asked him. Given how defensive he became, I acknowledged his feelings and suggested we examine them. This acknowledgement seemed to make Mr. Garcia less defensive, and he was able to become more reflective about the situation. When I observed his angry affect toward his son (who did not show much interest in him) and his willingness to be with and experience affection from his own father, Mr. Garcia was able to identify feeling rejected and unloved by his son. Mr. Garcia interpreted his son's response as being a blatant personal rejection. He viewed his son's refusal to go to the movies with him as meaning that his son did not care about or enjoy being with him.

As we explored his frustrations toward his son, it was quite surprising to learn that, despite Mr. Garcia's level of frustration and criticism of his son's deficits and problematic behaviors, he was unwilling to discipline him in times when he thought some consequence was necessary. After examining several situations in which these problems arose, it seemed that Mr. Garcia's difficulties with punishment were related to the physical abuse he experienced in his own childhood. In one of our later sessions, I made the interpretation that punishing his son must be difficult for him given the tight control and arbitrary abuse that his mother inflicted on him. While Mr. Garcia did not outwardly agree with this interpretation, he became quiet and seemed affected by it. In order to facilitate his ability to discuss this issue, I focused on acknowledging and empathizing with the pain that his mother's abuse had caused him. With this recognition, he was more able to explore the possibility that some type of strategy may be appropriate and even beneficial for his son. After this session, complaints about his son's defiant behavior seemed to lessen in frequency and intensity. Further, several sessions later, he reported that his son was being more compliant with rules he had put in place. He stated that it was still fairly difficult to implement certain types of behavioral management techniques, but was becoming better able to manage the anxiety related to his own experience.

On a number of occasions early in treatment, Mr. Garcia stated that he needed to talk about his sexuality, but this would occur at the end of a session, when there was clearly not enough time to address the issue. When I observed this pattern to him, he stated that I would need to force him to talk about it because he feared that I would judge or reject him. I reassured him that he could freely talk about any topic in therapy, including sexuality, and I would not judge him. However, this did not seem to alleviate his fears, as he still expressed great hesitancy to be open about this part of himself.

It should be noted here that his sexual comments at the end of the session were not the only manifestations of sexual conflict I saw in our sessions. Mr. Garcia demonstrated strong sexualized transference towards me, stating that I was attractive and accusing me on a few occasions of sexually seducing him when I brought up the topic of his sexual concerns. I viewed these comments as a projection, which represented more unconscious feelings of danger associated with his sexual arousal. Such feelings were very threatening to him, since he perceived me as someone who was incapable of understanding him, which, in this case, was part of his transference to me as a mother who could not and would not understand him.

As these issues arose more and more, I began to think about Mr. Garcia's sexual conflicts and how these might play out in our work together. His conflicts seemed to be characterized by the contrast of sadism and masochism. His heterosexual relationships were highly sadistic, often aimed at fulfilling his sexual and aggressive needs. He took pleasure in having control over women sexually and emotionally. For example, when describing his sexual experiences with women, he reported always having a desire to initiate sex. If these initiatives were not met, he would become extremely angry and hostile. He expected that women should always be willing to fulfill his sexual needs and submit completely to him. Quite interestingly, Mr. Garcia described himself in these situations as an exhibitionist, in that he requested women to perform sexual acts with him in public places. This, I believe, reflected desires to be viewed by others as sexually potent and powerful in a way that would leave no doubt in others' minds of his sexual appeal and masculinity (see below). In contrast, his homosexual experiences and fantasy life were more masochistic in nature. These experiences were always anonymous and often with older men. He would take on a very submissive role in these interactions, often being restrained or being told to perform sexual acts. He felt a strong sense of guilt and shame for finding so much pleasure in these activities. Not only were they sinful in terms of his religious beliefs, they directly contradicted his more conscious, "moral" heterosexual desires. However, from what I could assess at the time, they seemed to be representative of desires for care and nurturance from a father figure, who in this case was more interested in his needs and desires than those of his son.

The contrast between his sadistic heterosexual behaviors and his masochistic homosexual behaviors were clearly linked to his relationships with his mother and father. Mr. Garcia had a tendency to portray the people in his life as all-good or all-bad, and this was most clearly exemplified in his descriptions of his parents. He expressed profound hostility and aggression towards his mother. In recounting his interactions with her, he would ruminatively focus on her negative comments toward him or her lack of concern about him. He also expressed much criticism toward his mother's desire to be the center of attention. Though he expressed staunch refusal to give his mother the attention she attempted to elicit from others, he spent an inordinate amount of time and energy in his internal life obsessing and ruminating over her behaviors. Mr. Garcia's relationship with his mother elicited feelings of vulnerability and powerlessness. He felt that he had little control over his mother's abusive and dominating behavior. However, his sadistic heterosexual behaviors allowed him to avoid these negative feelings. He gained a sense of control and power over his mother by forcing other females to submit to him.

In contrast to his all-bad view of his mother, Mr. Garcia expressed a highly idealized view of his father. In Mr. Garcia's eyes, his father could do no wrong, which seemed much like the childish quality with which a young boy admires his father. When talking about his father, Mr. Garcia elicited a sense of helplessness and an infantile need for a father, but was unable to acknowledge the fact that his father could be neglectful or rejecting of him. Whenever problems arose in his relationship with his father, he would express great distress, and he would begin to feel hopeless about his future. Thus, Mr. Garcia's relationship with his father was likely played out in his masochistic homosexual tendencies: he would become submissive to an older man, which mirrored the power a father has over his son, but yet act in ways that only served to gratify the man and not him. By engaging in

these relationships, he was indirectly able to satisfy his fantasies of an idealized father and son relationship.

Mr. Garcia struggled with a strong need for the love and acceptance of
others while also having prominent desires for control and intense hostility towards others. This was exemplified in not only his relationship with
his parents, but also his relationship with his son. While he openly criticized and humiliated his son, his self-esteem was dependent on his son's affection and concern for him, as well as his ability to control his son's behavior. This was observed further in his career difficulties. When discussing
the professional problems that preceded the onset of his depression, Mr.
Garcia expressed a great degree of hostility toward other employees at his
company, most of whom were Caucasian. He stated that he felt better now
being out of the company, given all of the hypocrisy and unethical behavior he observed. However, he also struggled with feelings of worthlessness
as a result of not having job. This situation clearly exemplified Mr. Garcia's
conflict between being an autonomous individual, yet finding it hurtful to
be rejected by someone important to him. Further, this experience was reminiscent of his relationship with his mother. While he aggressively asserted
his independence from his mother, he unconsciously felt dependent on her
to meet his basic needs.

As issues about his mother and father entered our sessions more frequently, it was not surprising that Mr. Garcia's fear of abandonment also entered into the therapy relationship. At the 31st session, Mr. Garcia began to
express concerns that I would soon be transferring him to a new therapist. He
stated that he did not want to share any more personal information with me
until he could be certain that I would continue to treat him for at least another year. I explained that it would be difficult to guarantee how long I
would be able to treat him, but I did not have any immediate plans to transfer him in the next year. I then said that I felt it was important to explore from
where these concerns were originating, since when he perceives that he is becoming too emotionally involved, he leaves the relationship before he is left
by the other person. He denied that this pattern was an issue here, stating that
it was only a practical concern he had. He added that he did not want to
waste his time with me if I was just going to pass him on to someone else.

Despite his disinterest and defensiveness, it was clear that Mr. Garcia was
finding himself emotionally attached and did not want me to hurt him.
This fear mirrored his relationship with his mother and the various women
in his life. He felt that he could not trust me or continue to allow himself
to be vulnerable for fear that I would hurt him like his mother did. Like his
past romantic relationships, he felt a desire to end our relationship before
I ended it and caused him pain. I believed it was important for Mr. Garcia
to continue in treatment with me despite the ambiguity about how long the
therapeutic relationship would last. Consequently, I attempted to explore

the transference reaction in spite of his denial and resistance. Over several sessions, we examined how it felt to be vulnerable with me and what fears he has about what I might do to him. Because we had formed a strong therapeutic alliance by this point, Mr. Garcia gradually became able to openly explore these unconscious fears about me and how they relate to his relationship with his mother. For example, he came to recognize that his perception of my "abandoning" him in treatment would likely cause him emotional pain and convey the message that I did not care about him. These feelings would be very reminiscent of the feelings he felt when his mother abused him or neglected to protect him. After gaining greater insight into this issue, Mr. Garcia was better able to examine the distortion in these fears and beliefs, as well as manage his anxiety about abandonment.

Because of Mr. Garcia's tenuous sense of self and deep-seated insecurities, he projected a grandiose, inflated view of himself and acted in ways that would keep genuine interactions to a minimum. By doing this, he was able to avoid caring about others and thus avoid being hurt. He was also able to avoid having his self-esteem shattered if others said anything remotely critical or rejected him. However, despite the protective purpose of this mode of functioning, it was preventing him from developing healthy and adaptive interactions with others. The lack of appropriate interactions with others further caused Mr. Garcia to feel rejected and promoted his insecurities, which then in turn increased his need to project an inflated self-esteem.

After treating Mr. Garcia for about six months, I underwent a minor surgery and had to wear a bandage to session. I did not bring up the subject with Mr. Garcia and conducted the session as I normally would. However, about ten minutes into the session, he asked me what had happened. I very generally explained to him that I had had a minor surgery. He was quiet for a few seconds, and then expressed a desire for my prompt return to good health. This was the first time I ever witnessed Mr. Garcia express any degree of empathy toward another person. It seemed that seeing me, a person whom he had begun to idealize, accept my own faults and imperfections was therapeutic for him. The tolerance and acceptance I displayed toward my own difficulties acted as a model for him to tolerate his own faults. When he became less judgmental and more accepting of the fact that he was not perfect, he was better able to be empathetic toward others. His display of empathy could also be seen as a testament to the strong therapeutic alliance that we had developed. He was beginning to have more positive feelings towards me. As a result, I saw him act in a manner more consistent with these positive feelings, such as empathizing with me and being more trusting of me. This was in sharp contrast to his previous defensive and cold behaviors that were likely rooted in his poor sense of self and strong fear of abandonment. Even after this occurrence, Mr. Garcia continued to exhibit greater empathy and relatedness in our therapeutic interactions.

COUNTERTRANSFERENCE

Mr. Garcia was one of the first patients I saw during my practicum training. Thus, I was relatively inexperienced in providing psychotherapy. I lacked confidence in my ability to effectively implement clinical interventions with patients. When I accepted Mr. Garcia's case, I was aware that he would be challenging to treat. He had a history of being critical and mistrusting of clinicians. Further, he had already disclosed his concerns about my gender and ethnicity to his previous therapist. Thus, I was quite anxious about being able to build a therapeutic alliance and earn Mr. Garcia's trust. I met with my supervisor a number of times before seeing Mr. Garcia—a step I believed was crucial in lessening my anxiety and helping me feel more prepared for my first session with Mr. Garcia. My supervisor and I discussed my anxieties and identified how they may affect how Mr. Garcia perceives or responds to me. For example, I was very anxious that Mr. Garcia would try to challenge me. As a result, I was concerned that I would come off as defensive in light of my anxious feelings. With the help of my supervisor, I recognized in this situation that the focus should be on Mr. Garcia's concerns about me. In other words, I recognized I was there for him—to understand and make sense of his fears and concerns. There would be time later on—in supervision—to focus my attention on my reactions. Despite my preparation, I was still surprised by my first session with Mr. Garcia. His focus on my appearance made me feel objectified. I also felt that my professionalism was compromised.

Although this was a challenging case, it was a valuable training experience. As a beginning therapist, one is often so focused on performing psychotherapy "correctly" that our basic human instincts, such being empathic and considerate, can fall to the wayside. However, in the treatment of individuals with narcissistic traits, it is crucial to express understanding and respect. Not being genuine with patients or not providing them with support can have negative effects on the building of therapeutic rapport or could even cause them to prematurely terminate from therapy. However, to adequately provide patients with necessary support and empathy, it was important for me to work through my own countertransference reactions. This is especially important when treating patients with narcissistic personality disorder, since it is common to have negative or hostile countertransference reactions.

For instance, many times I felt myself becoming angry and frustrated with Mr. Garcia. His constant testing of my skills and ability to understand him often left me feeling frustrated and annoyed. It became important to discuss these reactions with my supervisor, as it helped me gain perspective into why Mr. Garcia felt the need to have me prove myself to him. Processing these reactions also allowed me to explore the effect that my negative emotional response may have had on my interactions with my patient or how my patient perceived me. For example, my frustration and annoyance could easily be expressed through my body language (e.g. crossing my arms, clenching my jaw). Thus, we discussed the importance of being very aware of my body language and what message it was conveying. If these negative reactions were not worked through, it was likely that Mr. Garcia would have easily noticed them and felt as though I was being too critical and rejecting.

I also found myself feeling demoralized and rejected by Mr. Garcia. This reaction most commonly occurred after he made comments about my professionalism and my appearance. As a beginning therapist, it is easy to feel insecure about how patients will perceive you. Because I was a relatively young student therapist and had had very little therapy experience, I was concerned that I would not be viewed as a professional. Recognizing these fears and discussing them with my supervisor, as well as with other student therapists, helped me to normalize and work through these insecurities. This helped me to feel and appear less anxious in sessions, which further improved my image of professionalism and sense of authority. For example, I was concerned that my patient would interpret my youthful appearance to mean that I was inexperienced or not able to understand his middle adulthood issues. However, through discussions with my supervisor and other student therapists, I internalized more fully that I have expertise, skills, and knowledge that will help patients. This realization helped me gain more confidence in the image I portray to patients.

Some other important countertransference reactions should be noted. During sessions with Mr. Garcia, I would often feel as if I were being ignored or was not even in the room with him. I had the sense that he would say the same things about himself regardless of whether I was there listening to him. Compounding this feeling was the fact that Mr. Garcia had a tendency not to acknowledge comments I would make or would avoid answering questions I asked. For example, he would frequently ignore the interpretations that I made to him. I believe that this tendency was a way to protect himself from feeling more insecure about himself or face the fact that he was disillusioning himself. However, even though I was able to identify reasons for his behavior, it often left me feeling helpless, as if he did not have respect for my authority or expertise. These ideas have been elaborated by many other, including McWilliams (1994) and Schultz and Glickhauf-Hughes (1995).

As therapy progressed, I found myself having less frustration and demoralized countertransference reactions. As my therapeutic alliance with Mr. Garcia strengthened, and he stopped doubting my competence, I found it easier to experience more genuine compassion toward him, which later shifted into vague rescue fantasies. However, these rescue fantasies were largely unconscious and were thus not easily recognizable. Following Mr.

Garcia's suicide threat, I felt more positive toward him, in that it was at this point that he allowed me to see behind his callous and demeaning exterior. I began to see him more as someone who was very insecure and troubled, and began to provide him with increasing amounts of support and praise. Unconsciously, I believed that if I formed a good enough relationship with him and showed him the concern that he was never shown when he was a child, he would be able to work through his conflicts and have his narcissistic needs satisfied. I did not recognize these unconscious motives until my supervisor suggested that I begin to "push" Mr. Garcia out of his comfort zone a bit. After the supervisor suggested this, I was instinctively opposed to it. This ran counter to my unconscious belief that Mr. Garcia would be "healed" if I showed him enough concern and compassion.

After recognizing these ideas, I discussed them with my supervisor and watched some of my taped sessions to observe how these fantasies were playing themselves out. This was quite helpful. In fact, watching videos of myself in session was particularly useful in managing my countertransference reactions. While I would try my best to be aware of my emotional responses to my patient, it was often difficult to recognize how these reactions played out in body language and verbal communication. For example, I observed that I often was too apologetic for fairly minor things (e.g. a phone ringing during session, needing to cancel a session due to illness). After becoming aware of this behavior, I was able to more closely monitor and avoid it.

One thing that made working with this patient especially difficult was his constant, overriding need to impress others with power, wealth, knowledge, and/or attractiveness. Narcissistic patients' choices and behaviors exemplify their feeling that validation of their sense of self is their most important need. They destroy relationships with friends or family, keep others at a distance, take advantage of others, and break down others' self-worth. This is all done in an effort to impress the world with superficial signs of success. At face value, this can cause therapists to have a very negative response, since the patients' criteria for evaluating themselves contradicts the self-evaluation criteria the therapist holds. Alternatively, the need felt by the patient to impress others with external criteria may stimulate the clinician's unconscious shame about their own unrecognized narcissism (McWilliams, 1994).

Regardless of what effect patients' pull for external recognition has, it is important that these feelings are recognized and worked through in supervision. To facilitate this work, it consequently may be useful to review the values and manner by which one's own self-esteem is derived. If one realizes that his or her values are vastly different from the values or narcissistic needs of the patient, it may be necessary to transfer the patient to a clinician whose values are more moderate or are more tolerant to the needs of the narcissist. As pointed out by McWilliams (1994), if the clinician and the patient are too divergent in their values, the clinician's empathy may remain unaccessed. For example, if a clinician treating Mr. Garcia has strong moral objections to homosexuality, their empathic understanding of Mr. Garcia's sexual conflicts may be greatly impaired. The *patient* may also have difficulty therapeutically if their self-esteem requirements are vastly different from the clinicians. To assess this, McWilliams (1994) recommends that clinicians examine their own countertransference reactions to the patient's behaviors and expressed values, as well as be aware of how their own values may run counter to the patient's and affect the way the patient is able to benefit from the therapeutic relationship. Even if the countertransference reactions are worked through and deemed not to impair treatment, one should monitor transference reactions to ensure that they are not impairing the effects of therapy.

I frequently found the countertransference reactions I had to be surprising and somewhat distressing, as they were largely out of character for me. As a person who enjoys working with people and prides herself on her ability to listen and be empathic to others' experiences, I began to worry that my skills may not have been as strong as I once thought. I also became concerned that my patient was causing me to become calloused. For example, I found myself becoming bored in session and would frequently complain to my supervisor about the monotony of sessions. My supervisor reassured me that these were frequent complaints by therapists treating narcissistic patients. In addition, he suggested readings about narcissistic personality disorder (e.g. Gabbard, 2005; Kernberg, 1975, 1976, 1984; Kohut, 1968, 1971, 1977 McWilliams, 1999; Schultz and Glickhauf-Huges, 1995) that helped me gain insight into possible reasons why I was having these countertransference reactions.

I found discussing countertransference reactions in the context of group supervision in addition to individual supervision to be very useful. The other student therapists in group supervision had not watched videotapes of the patient, which minimized their potential for bias that could have occurred due to knowledge of his in-session behaviors. Other student therapists were able to normalize my experience or give me advice on how to work through the reactions. They were also able to share their experiences of how countertransference reactions affected the outcome of their therapeutic work.

Discussing my countertransference reactions in individual and group supervision also provided me with ideas about when and how countertransference should be recognized and utilized therapeutically. For example, Mr. Garcia used to report that acquaintances at church would act as if they were annoyed by him or would appear bored when he was talking to them. Further, he sensed that they did not know how to respond to him. When we

explored the content of his conversations with these acquaintances, it became clear to me that Mr. Garcia would relentlessly talk about himself and
his accomplishments and would allow them very little time to ask him
questions or respond to him. However, while this was readily apparent to
me, Mr. Garcia had little insight into his effect on others.

After discussing this observation with my supervisor, I was advised to utilize my countertransference reactions to determine what behavioral observations I should bring to Mr. Garcia's attention. I explained to Mr. Garcia
that, while he is encouraged to speak about himself in session, I found that
he often fixates on talking about his accomplishments and signs of his success. I then asked him if he acts similarly when he talks with his acquaintances as church. While at first he was resistant to the idea that he had a tendency to focus on himself, he began to entertain it and reported that his
interactions with me are fairly similar to his interactions with others in his
life. I then asked him how he might feel if someone he was talking to spoke
only about their successes and did not ask him any questions or allow him
to respond to what they had to say. He stated that he would probably feel
irritated and would want to stop talking to that person. We then related this
to the way he reported his acquaintances were reacting to him. By being
cognizant of my countertransference reactions, I was able to gain insight
into why individuals in Mr. Garcia's life responded to him in a negative
manner. Further, I was able to point this out to Mr. Garcia, without directly
identifying that this was the way I was feeling, which could have negatively
affected the therapeutic alliance.

Especially as a beginning therapist, it can be highly intimidating to treat
a patient with narcissistic personality disorder. Because of their deep-seated
insecurities, it is difficult for narcissistic patients to ask for help from someone who may be perceived as more successful or intelligent than them.
Therefore, they may attempt to assert their superiority over the clinician. Mr.
Garcia, for instance, had a history of seeking treatment at training clinics.
While he never explicitly stated his reasons for choosing training clinics, he
was more than able to afford treatment from a fully licensed provider. My
supervisor and I thought that being seen by a student may have allowed
him to feel more superior in the relationship. There was less of a power and
status differential that could have potentially caused him to feel even more
insecure about himself.

In treating patients with narcissistic personality disorder, therapists also
should examine their expectations about treatment and the therapeutic alliance. For example, I was somewhat naïve in my thinking that I would be
"the one person" to form a strong alliance with Mr. Garcia and finally help
him work through his conflicts. I expected to be able to provide him with
the compassion and understanding he needed but was never given. However, after a few months of treatment, I felt as if I was not able to give him

as much support as I had thought. No matter how much I provided, he continued to demand more. It was at that point that I realized that it is virtually impossible to avoid disappointing these individuals, as it is almost inevitable that any therapist will fall short of their patient's unrealistic demands for validation and praise.

Even despite the virtual impossibility to providing patients with narcissistic personality disorder with the amount of support that they often demand, providing empathic validation is a crucial component in the treatment of these patients. I became aware of this fact early on in treatment when Mr. Garcia both covertly and overtly questioned my willingness to understand him and not judge him. This distrust impaired our ability to build good therapeutic report, and prevented Mr. Garcia from discussing topics that had great importance in his life but made him feel vulnerable. However, as treatment progressed and I expressed greater empathic validation, the tension in our therapeutic relationship dissipated greatly and Mr. Garcia became less resistant of talking about these difficult issues.

For a significant period in the beginning of my treatment with Mr. Garcia, I felt as if the therapeutic alliance was very tenuous. Regardless of how much I worked to cultivate the therapeutic rapport, I felt as if, at any moment, he would terminate treatment. After discussing this perception with my supervisor and reading more about narcissistic personality, I began to understand more about why I felt this way. While Mr. Garcia demanded much from the therapeutic relationship, he appeared to contribute very little to it. He had an expectation that I, as the provider, would do most of the work. This expectation left me feeling as if the therapeutic relationship was one-sided. For instance, I came to see that I was the one who was most hopeful for Mr. Garcia by expecting that treatment would alleviate his distress. However, Mr. Garcia conveyed a lack of motivation and did not seem to have faith in his ability to overcome his problems. At times, this perception of the relationship was very frustrating and left me feeling helpless. However, by understanding how it related to Mr. Garcia's pathology and how it played on some of my insecurities, I became more comfortable with the ambiguity that surrounded the therapeutic alliance. This helped me become less fearful that making interpretations about Mr. Garcia's behavior or confronting his defense mechanisms would lead to him prematurely terminating from treatment.

During sessions with Mr. Garcia, I would often feel as if I were being ignored or was not even in the room with him. I had the sense that he would say the same things about himself regardless of whether I was there listening to them. Compounding this feeling was the fact that Mr. Garcia had a tendency not to acknowledge comments I would make or would avoid answering questions I asked. For example, he would frequently ignore the interpretations that I made to him. I believe that this tendency was a way to protect himself from feeling more insecure about himself or face the fact that he was disillusioning himself. However, even though I was able to identify reasons for his behavior, it often left me feeling helpless, as if he did not have respect for my authority or expertise.

If I were to provide some advice for therapists treating patients with narcissistic personality disorder, I would recommend constantly remaining aware of your expectations for the outcome of treatment. Providing psychotherapy to these patients is often slow and arduous, and requires patience on the part of the therapist. If the goals of treatment are too lofty or on a short-lived time frame, it is likely that the therapist will feel discouraged or frustrated. Further, if expectations of progress or goals are not realistic, it may be easy to lose sight of what the overall objectives in treatment are. To help moderate one's expectations for treatment, it is important to discuss goals with both the patient and your supervisor. It may also be useful to consult the literature to gain more information about what can be realistically expected in terms of outcomes.

SUMMARY

This chapter has presented my experiences in the treatment of a patient with a highly prototypical presentation of narcissistic personality disorder. Throughout therapy, Mr. Garcia presented with strong themes of victimization and a fear of abandonment. In the context of the therapeutic relationship, he was highly mistrusting of me and often devaluing. Over the course of treatment, my countertransference reactions ranged from boredom to hostility to rescue fantasies. Further, all of these countertransference reactions had an intense, consuming characteristic (McWilliams, 1994, Schultz & Glickhauf-Huges, 1995). My clinical work with Mr. Garcia was a highly enlightening experience.

NOTES

1. I would like to express my appreciation and thankfulness to the following individuals who served as supervisors on this case: Norman Gordon PhD, Flora Hoodin PhD, and Ellen Koch PhD.

2. Despite his frustration about discontinuing treatment with his former therapist, Mr. Garcia did sign a release for me to speak with the former therapist.

REFERENCES

Gabbard, G. O. (2005). *Psychodynamic psychiatry in clinical practice*. Washington, DC: American Psychiatric Publishing Inc.

Kernberg, O. (1975). *Borderline conditions and pathological narcissism.* New York, NY: Jason Aronson.

Kernberg, O. (1976). *Object relations theory and clinical psychoanalysis.* New York, NY: Jason Aronson.

Kernberg, O. (1984). *Severe personality disorders: Psychotherapeutic strategies.* New Haven, CT: Yale University Press.

Kohut, H. (1968). The psychoanalytic treatment of narcissistic personality disorders: Outline of a systematic approach. *The Psychoanalytic Study of the Child, 23,* 86–113.

Kohut, H. (1971). *The analysis of the self: A systematic approach to the psychoanalytic treatment of narcissistic personality disorders.* New York: International Universities Press.

Kohut, H. (1977). *The restoration of the self.* New York: International Universities Press.

McWilliams, N. (1994). *Psychoanalytic diagnosis.* New York: Guilford

McWilliams, N. (1999). *Psychoanalytic case formulation.* New York: Guilford.

Schultz, R. E. & Glickauf-Hughes, C. (1995). Countertransference in the treatment of pathological narcissism. *Psychotherapy, 32,* 601–07.

4

The Case of Mr. Miller

J. Robert Parker[1]

CASE DESCRIPTION

Mr. Miller was a twenty-six-year-old male who was referred to therapy following a suicide attempt. He presented himself as a tough, street-wise individual with several tattoos, long dark hair, and often wore dark sunglasses, chains, and a leather jacket. Mr. Miller was diagnosed with Major Depressive Disorder, but it became increasingly evident as time progressed that he had a narcissistic personality. Consistent with Gabbard (2003), Mr. Miller's narcissism was comprised of a mixture of the overt and covert types (see Wink, 1991). Primarily, he displayed introversion, defensiveness, and a particular vulnerability and aversion to the normal traumatic events of life that characterize covert narcissism, as well as the aggression and some degree of the exhibitionism that are indicative of overt narcissism. Specifically, he demonstrated a tendency to embellish stories of his actions or life events in terms that were quite graphic, frequently difficult to believe, and best described as fitting for a video game or action movie.

Prior to entering therapy, Mr. Miller described himself as playing the role of the "hero," which referred to his tendency to help and save people from all sorts of danger situations or potential attacks. Additionally, he was prone to outbursts of anger and aggressive behavior, having been involved in several arguments and physical altercations over the years. Indicative of his more covert narcissistic traits, he had been deeply affected by deaths of family members and friends, as well as being the victim of childhood bullying, which had instilled in him a deep fear of distress and sadness, and an intense avoidance of emotion and emotionally difficult events. He was quite distrustful of the motives of others and was prone to perceiving personal threats in their actions.

In his paper on character pathology, Kernberg (1970) notes that many individuals with narcissistic traits display behavior that is indicative of a notably undeveloped ego and superego, which are unable to fully counteract the strongly impulsive nature of the id. In such individuals, there is an inability to feel empathy for others, over-reliance on immature defenses (such as splitting and denial), an inability to withstand ambiguity within people or situations, and vivid fantasies of power, wealth, influence, and even veneration. More severe cases even show evidence of paranoid ideation, and are differentiated from psychotic symptoms primarily by the level of the patient's reality testing. Mr. Miller demonstrated several of these traits. For instance, he demonstrated black-and-white thinking on many issues (splitting), which was captured by his representations of family, friends, and enemies. He also demonstrated an aversion to emotional experience, in that he believed experiencing any negative emotion would immediately result in feeling overwhelmed and being unable to cope effectively with them. There was no room in his mind for tolerable experiences of negative emotion. Moreover, even positive emotions were threatening because they would eventually dissipate, and he would have to resume feeling other, more painful feelings, which in turn would overwhelm him. Therefore, with the exception of anger, emotions of all kinds were "bad," and only the absence of emotion was acceptable. He often expressed a deep distrust of others and concern that people would try to manipulate or take advantage of him, and he was very prone to describing himself in grandiose, even fantastical, terms.

Therapy developed steadily and lasted for a period of over two years. He attended weekly sessions that were primarily psychodynamic in nature, though we occasionally incorporated other techniques, such as cognitive-behavioral interventions. Though we addressed Mr. Miller's characterological issues throughout therapy, treatment could be divided into roughly two phases. The first phase addressed his depression specifically, while the second addressed his characterological structure in general. The shift from the first phase to the second began when he acknowledged that his depressive symptoms had remitted, but believed that he continued to have issues that troubled him. More specifically, he often described himself as emotionally dead, explaining that most emotions were something he avoided because they were simply too painful—that they were parts of his experience that clouded his judgment, and kept him from thinking clearly about how to solve his problems. As noted earlier, the only emotion that Mr. Miller readily recognized or acknowledged was an ever-present sense of anger. This was something that was always just under the surface, and something that would quickly rise and fuel significant, often physically violent, responses to whatever may have triggered his anger.

BACKGROUND AND DEVELOPMENT

Mr. Miller was the middle of three children, all of whom grew up with their parents in a lower-middle-class suburb of a large Midwestern city. At the time of his therapy, he was the only child still living at home, while his older sister had married and moved across the country, and his younger brother lived on campus at a local university. Mr. Miller was a student at a community college while working part-time at a gas station. His father was a moderately successful small-business owner, and his mother worked as a secretary and bookkeeper for his father's business.

Mr. Miller described his relationships with his parents as generally loving and supportive, though there were periods of tension that occurred throughout his adolescence and early adulthood. He frequently described how alike he and his father were, especially identifying with his father's stubbornness and temper, and difficulty controlling their tempers when provoked. Additionally, each one was adamant that things be done in his way. When their ideas collided, verbal conflict was likely to occur as neither one was likely to capitulate. Mr. Miller also identified with his father in another way—both he and his father had a physical disability. Mr. Miller's father has lost the use of a limb as the result of an industrial accident as a young man. Despite this disability, his father was able to become quite successful at a number of activities which normally require considerable physical skill. Mr. Miller was born with a slightly deformed foot, making it difficult for him to walk with a smooth gait. Yet, he too was able to be quite successful in a number of his own interests, despite his own disability. This fact further strengthened Mr. Miller's "super-hero" identification with of his father, who could overcome weakness and act in powerful and resourceful ways.

Mr. Miller's relationship with his mother was less often openly contentious. He often idealized her, and especially her ability to know what advice or course of action would be the most beneficial for him. Throughout the therapy, he often spoke of her as being the only person who really knew him well. Even at twenty-six years old, he suggested that his mother have access to his files and information from therapy, if this could be helpful to treatment.[2] At the same time, he expressed considerable frustration with the notion that she was "always right," interpreting this as meaning that she knew him better than he knew himself. As such, he developed a strong degree of ambivalence toward her, expressing his alternating love and frustration with his mother in black-and-white terms. It appeared to me that, despite his strong desire to maintain control over his life and make his own choices, Mr. Miller felt little confidence in his actual ability to do so effectively. This introduced yet another degree of ambivalence, not toward his mother per se, but toward himself, which further reinforced my assessment of his conflict (i.e., he outwardly promoted a persona of control and competence, while inwardly experiencing little self-efficacy). His desire to include her in his treatment indicated some awareness of his inability to maintain self control and make effective decisions for himself. Also, it signaled some reluctance on his part to fully invest himself in a process that would ultimately require him to accept his current difficulty and make significant changes. Even the fact that he continued to live at home, despite frequent protestations that he was more than able to take care of himself, provided additional evidence to support this ambivalence.

As a part of their parenting beliefs, Mr. Miller's parents often refrained from open displays of emotion in front of their children. He recalled some physical and verbal expressions of love and support from his mother, but far less from his father. In the case of more negative emotions, neither parent openly displayed their feelings. Mr. Miller explained on a number of occasions that his parents refrained from such displays out of a desire to protect their children from pain or confusion. By his recollection, their reasoning was that if a child were to see his/her parents visibly upset, in pain, or confused, it would only upset, confuse, and scare the child. The parents' limited displays of negative emotion were characterized mostly by anger and by a loss of temper. Mr. Miller's father was particularly prone to this, which considerably affected Mr. Miller's understanding of emotional regulation and experience. Consequently, as Mr. Miller became older, he learned that it would be his responsibility to protect others from seeing his own emotions, just as his parents had protected him. This was perhaps the beginning of a "hero" identity that he displayed so openly in his later adolescent years and early twenties. As he was taught that emotions were dangerous and was protected from them by his parents, he began to take on an exaggerated version of this role, working to protect all of those for whom he cared from the negative experiences of life, and especially from the pain and confusion that seeing him experience emotion would cause.

Mr. Miller's disability influenced his development in ways other than his identification with his father. Throughout his time in grade school, he was teased and humiliated by other children on a frequent basis. During these incidents, his disability was most often the target of the teasing, and he referred to them as "torture." After being subjected to such teasing for several years, he learned to fight and present a "tough guy" image with the hope that others would leave him alone. Additionally, he sought refuge in books, movies, and video games that presented a protagonist who often suffered some sort of injustice and who protected others from similar problems, often by violent, aggressive means. He began to identify very strongly with these characters and the virtues that they fought to uphold, including independence, decisiveness, a personal sense of honor and integrity, and especially a sense of being the wronged avenger. The games also served as a defensive mechanism by allowing him to escape the real-life difficulties that he experienced and immerse himself in a world where he was in more control over events and could affect the outcomes of situations in much more tangible ways than he was experiencing in his daily life.

During his life, Mr. Miller experienced the illness and death of several family members and friends, and it was this set of events with which he was most preoccupied. Atop these losses was the death of his paternal grandmother, when he was twelve years old. Mr. Miller had spent much of his life with his grandmother in various family functions and was quite attached to her. Her death was the first significant loss that he recalled. Interestingly, what was most powerful to him about this experience was seeing his father cry and grieve openly for the first time at the funeral. Up until this time in his life, Mr. Miller maintained an image of his father as a type of near-superhero. He recalled how he was entirely unprepared to witness "human weakness" in his father. His father, who had always protected him from the pain and confusion that would surely come with such sadness, had failed to protect himself and his son now when needed most. At seeing this display from his father, Mr. Miller had "a complete breakdown." He began to sob uncontrollably and only vaguely recalled what he was later told by his family; that he collapsed in the church and was so inconsolable that he had to be carried out. Mr. Miller recalled being so scared and disturbed by his own reaction that he decided he would never again experience such deep sadness and despair.

This set of experiences served to strengthen his tendencies to glorify aggressive and violent behavior as a proper approach to solving problems, and to see himself as a protector of others. During my first session with Mr. Miller, he told me a series of stories from his late teens and early twenties in which he literally saved others from terrible events, such as rape and mugging, by chasing down and fighting off attackers. An interesting aspect of Mr. Miller's discussions of his violent behaviors was that he was both proud and afraid of his "ability to fight." In his stories, he described himself as often losing control and blacking out, only to be pulled away from his opponent by friends who got there in the nick of time to keep him from seriously injuring or killing someone. Despite the dramatic and horrific nature of his stories, they were often untenable. Many of the events he described would have likely been investigated by police, yet there was never any report of legal trouble. He deflected any question of his having done these things without being questioned by police by simply being "lucky." Such stories strengthened my impression that they were a self-aggrandizing embellishment to which strongly narcissistic individuals are often prone. They also served the purpose of defending against the lack of confidence in his ability to make good choices about his life.

As in the case of his feelings about his mother, Mr. Miller was conflicted about the image he tried to present and the abilities he claimed to have. He strove to achieve a sense of grandiosity while being aware that the actions he claimed were generally only appropriate or rewarded in fiction. One of his most frequent statements during the first phases of therapy was, "I am not afraid of anything, except what I am capable of."

TREATMENT HISTORY

Treatment with Mr. Miller progressed relatively slowly and steadily. The first phase of treatment was spent addressing a large number of depressive symptoms, potential suicidality, and a persistent belief that his life was not worth anything. His depression was demonstrated by a very flat affect, persistent withdrawal from friends and family, strong feelings of guilt at his inability to stop pain and sadness in others, and sadness for himself at what he perceived to be a life not worth living. As he became aware that he could not "save" those for whom he cared from their own painful emotions, he began to have suicidal ideations. He also explained he had experienced a growing frustration with people whom he believed were only interested in him because of what he could do for them, and not out of any inherent interest in his own well-being. These thoughts combined to increase his feelings of worthlessness. He often stated that he considered life a "cruel joke" and that during his darkest periods he believed it was not worth living.

While the early diagnosis of Major Depression was easily reached within the first sessions or two, the detection of his narcissistic tendencies took a few session to identify. As his overt depressive symptoms began to decline, the pattern of painting himself as a tragic hero began to emerge and was the first strong indication of a narcissistic personality. This tragic hero role was one that Mr. Miller used to engage himself in the problems of all who surrounded him, personally investing himself in their solutions as a defense against facing his own distress. This was done even when there was not a way in which he could realistically help others. We explored this tendency, its origins, and its purpose because it was strongly related both to his depression and characterological issues. As Mr. Miller's mood and day-to-day functioning improved, he spent less and less time and energy engaging in this behavior and began to focus more intentionally on addressing his own needs. Before therapy, he was not well aware that his tendency to engage himself in others' problems was a way to distract himself from his own distress. As his awareness increased, however, his narcissistic qualities were manifested in a more classical sense. He began ignoring the impact he made on others as he sought to address his own issues, and he developed a more openly concerned, and even occasionally suspicious, attitude about the impact others would have on him.

The theme demonstrated earliest in Mr. Miller's treatment, which formed the basis of his narcissistic conflict, and which was the primary focus of therapy, was emotional avoidance and control. He worked diligently to maintain control of his emotions by suppressing them and avoiding any experience of them. He was quite intelligent, very introspective, and took pride in his intellectual abilities. These qualities made him a particularly good candidate for dynamic, insight-oriented therapy. He was very capable and willing to do the work, and he participated quite fully. However, he also frequently used his intellectualization as a defense to shift any uncomfortable focus off of himself in session. When asked about what he felt, he often described how people in general should feel in the situation in question, as opposed to how he actually felt. He spoke abstractly about the experience of emotion, as though it were something applied as an afterthought to the memory of an event to help one make more sense of what it meant, instead of being a part of the actual experience of the event. When pressed to apply these abstractions specifically to himself, he often became very uncomfortable, rapidly changing the subject to some tangential event that occurred during the week. Most often these events were ones that were frustrating to him and provoked some kind of angry response. His focus on an angry response allowed him to discuss his emotions in a much safer way than he otherwise could. Additionally, he enjoyed engaging in rather intellectualized discussions about the philosophical nature of emotions, especially love, hopefulness, and other positive emotions with which he was least comfortable.

Typically, Mr. Miller used intellectualization as a primary defense in all aspects of his life, not just in therapy. His pride in his intellect was particularly strong, and it was during times that he expounded on his logic for acting in a given way that he was most prone to grandiose statements about his ability to function in a crisis. However, he used intellectualization most frequently to defend against emotional experience. That is, while he slowly became willing to acknowledge the existence of his own emotions, and began to recall what he might have been feeling during past experiences, he was very reluctant to allow himself any emotional experience in the therapy room. For instance, he spoke of how being emotional could cloud his judgment and ability to act, that he typically acted as "a purely logical, unfeeling machine," and that others around him came to see him as the proverbial "anchor in a storm." Mr. Miller believed that his friends and family had become so accustomed to his lack of emotional expression that if he allowed himself to experience, and therefore express, any emotion apart from anger, they would take it as a sign that things were terribly wrong. In this way he maintained a very strong belief in his own importance to others and his ability to affect their lives. He also believed that if he became emotional, not only would he be unable to function and cope with his distress, but those around him would also be overwhelmed and unable to cope.

Though the extent of his narcissistic traits did not become evident until after the first several sessions, there was plenty of evidence that his depression was exacerbated by certain personality traits that needed immediate attention. For example, his need to prove his worth by protecting others and himself from painful emotions, but his inability to do so, gave him strong feelings of worthlessness and guilt. Whenever someone close to him was in distress that he could not alleviate, he interpreted this to mean that he was deficient and worthless. This not only increased his depressed mood, but also increased his internal conflict because he could not tolerate the idea that he could not do something so important.

Part of the difficulty I encountered during the first phase of therapy with Mr. Miller was due to two tendencies indicative of lower-level (i.e., more maladaptation) character pathology (Kernberg, 1970). The first of these was that he had a propensity to engage in splitting, seeing many things in terms of extremes. This was especially true of his understanding of how emotion is experienced. To Mr. Miller, there were only two types of emotional experiences. With the exception of anger, which was acceptable, he felt nothing at all or he became so consumed with distressing emotions that he felt overwhelmed and unable to cope with them. He acted as though there was no such thing as a pleasant emotion, and the only acceptable alternative to all-consuming distress was to suppress and deny the emotional effect that the events of life had on him. Interestingly, even anger was not entirely exempt from this belief. While he admitted feeling various degrees of anger, he had reported occasions when he became so angry that he was not able to cope with it either, and essentially "blacked out," unable to recall what happened. He remained fearful of this extreme degree of anger throughout his treatment.

Mr. Miller worked so hard to suppress his emotions that he was unable to recognize many negative emotions apart from anger. Therefore, one of the first tasks of early therapy was to help him differentiate emotions besides anger. As Mr. Miller discussed the times he felt provoked and angry, we worked slowly to identify thoughts, physical sensations, and other cues that indicated the presence of other affect. This was accomplished mainly through empathic validation and mirroring, with some explanation of the affect I observed as necessary. During these sessions, he began to recognize his emotions for what they were much more easily. These techniques presented him with an alternative to his parents' form of emotional instruction. He was shown that experiencing his emotions was not something inherently dangerous or made him weak, but was a normal and healthy human experience. In many ways my role became to "re-parent" him in the experiencing of his feelings.

These techniques also helped him to make sense of the multiple emotions he experienced, but which he had never been able to parse apart or cope with. He realized that whenever he was being threatened by something, he felt scared or anxious. As his previous experiences with such emotions were difficult to understand and often associated with traumatic events (such as the death of his grandmother), that lack of understanding and confusion led to an inability to process and cope with them, which became very confusing and frustrating. Unconsciously, part of this anger was directed toward himself for feeling scared and anxious in the first place. Another part of his anger was at others, or at the situations themselves, for the effects they had on him. His anger also served a similar protective function, in that when his confusion and frustration were no longer containable, they were vented in the form of anger.

The second character-organization quality I observed in Mr. Miller was his propensity towards a life filled with crisis and turmoil. Each week, almost without fail, a friend or family member would have some difficulty, and Mr. Miller would insert himself into that person's affairs, taking a very personal stake in the outcome and in his ability to influence them. It was in these events that his "hero" persona was used most often; he spoke at length throughout a number of sessions about how important it was to him "to protect those who cannot protect themselves." As he tried to intervene in these situations, he also worked hard to suppress the experience of any emotion he felt within himself.

Another area that was suggestive of Mr. Miller's narcissistic conflict was his sex life, though throughout most of therapy he was rather hesitant to discuss it. Early on, any time that this subject came up he became very quiet and uncomfortable, rarely giving more than cursory answers and changing the subject. Even as therapy progressed and he became more willing to discuss it in general terms, he continued to display a certain hesitance to address it in any detail. For example, each week, patients in the treatment clinic where he was seen are required to complete a forty-five-item questionnaire that assesses the severity of any symptoms, their activity level, and their satisfaction with various aspects of their lives. When responding to the question "I have an unfulfilling sex life," Mr. Miller rarely ever responded with the provided options (which ranged in a Likert format from "Never" to "Almost Always"), and instead wrote in his own response of "Not Applicable." Early in his treatment, he explained that a woman to whom he had some attraction did not necessarily reciprocate his feelings, but would flirt with him in a way he described alternately as pleasurable and torturing. He maintained a strong interest in her for several weeks, often interacting with her despite openly acknowledging that he did not believe the relationship would develop further. Later, he was asked about an evening that he had spent with her. He would only reply that it was "a long night."

Two to three sessions after this event was brought up, he became comfortable enough to discuss his ideas about sex in a general sense, explaining that he maintained a high sense of integrity and honor, and never discussed with anyone what he and his partners did. He considered it completely private business. He reluctantly revealed that he and this woman had engaged in sexual activity, but discussed the event no further. Mr. Miller's reticence to discuss his sex life was suggestive of further narcissistic conflict; as he identified quite strongly with a traditionally strong masculine character, which ostensibly would include an active sex life, his discomfort in discussing it could be taken as suggestive of a discrepancy between the image he wished to project and the reality of his sex life. By cloaking his reticence in terms of privacy, dignity, and honor, he could continue to "protect" himself and others, maintain his image as the tough guy and hero, and avoid the discomfort of revealing (either to me or to himself) any distressing emotion he might have felt at such an admission.

Later in therapy, he became more comfortable with discussing the topic, and revealed that he was particularly interested in "bondage-dominance-sadism-masochism (BDSM). Interestingly, he explained that this interest had helped him understand himself better because of its organization around explicitly submissive and dominant roles. Typically, he equated a submissive role (not just sexually, but in life in general) to being made less than equal, perhaps even less than human, compared to others. In BDSM activities, he explained that he would partake in dominant or submissive roles. Yet, he noted that the submissive person actually has control in BDSM activities due to his/her use of "safe words," and that the control within the dominant role was really illusory. He noted that he still preferred the feeling of being in the dominant role, even if the control was an illusion. Yet, as I thought about these activities, I suspected that he very much wanted to experience interpersonal relationships in ways in which he could be in a more submissive role, yet feel safe. In essence, his sexual life suggested how difficult it was for him to enter into mutually *interdependent* relationships.

It is important to note that a prominent feature of the narcissistic personality is the tendency to perceive many incidents in life as intentional threats or insults, and to perceive them as being of larger import than they really are. During multiple sessions, Mr. Miller revealed that he felt he had to be constantly alert for those who would take advantage of or threaten him, or would take advantage of those for whom he cared. As this topic was addressed, it became increasingly evident that he was not concerned with the well-being of those close to him for their own sakes, but about the possibility of what impact harm to one of these people would have on him. He cared about others because, in part, he had learned that others could have an effect on him. Mr. Miller believed that this tendency grew out of his experiences of being teased and bullied in grade school, where others' comments engendered a sense that they were exercising some degree of power and malice over him. As we explored this idea further, Mr. Miller identified that, during the year prior to entering treatment, he was being manipulated into providing favors (such as gas or rides) for a couple of individuals. Though the nature of the things he provided for these people seemed harmless enough, his perception of the events was that their intent was malicious, and that he felt weak because he was unable to anticipate their intentions. His distress over being teased, manipulated, and being unable to entirely prevent these experiences culminated in his suicide attempt, and finally his reluctant entrance into treatment.

Another strong indicator of a narcissistic personality is a need to convince both oneself and others of the individual's perfection, superiority, or general lack of weakness. Such individuals often project a persona that is quite the opposite of what is felt or feared internally in order to convince others and the self that there are no internal characteristics that could be perceived as negative. This was most obvious when Mr. Miller exhibited his image as a streetwise tough guy, but admitted in session that this was only a disguise to keep others from knowing his fears and insecurities. Another particularly strong manifestation of this trait that emerged was Mr. Miller's need to be in total control of his emotions and any event that might evoke negative emotions. In fact, it became evident that this need for control was at the heart of his narcissistic conflict. Mr. Miller first discussed this need to be in control in rather grandiose and philosophical terms by referring to it as a love of free will. He believed that it was only right that he should be able to think and act as he saw fit, regardless of what others would have him think or do. This extended to his emotional life as well, and he began to see the experience of emotion as a sign of weakness; if he could not control his emotions, he was not acting according to his will, but was being manipulated by forces outside his control. To counter this, he had developed a self-image of high intelligence, competence in distress, and his "hero" persona. Any emotional experience that he was unable to turn on and off at will was in conflict with this self-image and reminded him of this perceived internal weakness. Emotions became things to be conquered because they stood in the way of his free will and ability to control his life. In this way, not only were the negative emotions themselves upsetting, but the fact that they had any effect on him greatly upset him as well.

Several sessions were spent focusing upon the nature of emotions, Mr. Miller's ideas about free will and control, and whether or not emotions were something that could be controlled. Cognitive techniques were used to explore his beliefs about what different emotions signified to him. Dynamic techniques were effective at helping him gain insight into why many of his strong emotions could be elicited by seemingly small events, and why having free will and choice were such important ideas to him. Throughout his treatment he retained a considerable degree of reluctance to engage in emotional experience, though as time went on he was less likely to deny their effects on him. He also began to retroactively assess his experiences in more realistic ways, and was able to be more comfortable with the idea of having experienced emotions after-the-fact, even though the notion of experiencing them in any present sense was difficult to accept.

Even more so, focusing on everyone else's problems protected Mr. Miller from the distress that would inevitably accompany the facing his own problems. It took some time for him to become comfortable exploring the patterns in his behavior and thinking before he was able to recognize his emotional experiences. Foremost among these issues was the fact that he had not allowed himself to acknowledge the pain and feeling of loss that came with the death of his grandmother, nor had he allowed himself to grieve for the deaths of another family member's infant child or of a friend his own age. Over the course of several sessions, he talked about the experience of his grandmother's death and funeral. He began to realize the degree to which he had internalized his parents' message that negative emotions were painful and should be avoided, and as he explored this idea, he realized how damaging it had become to suppress his feelings. Also, the more we discussed the impact that his grandmother's death had on him, the more he realized how sad he still felt, and after fourteen years he finally allowed himself to grieve. Finally, he began to realize that some of his distress was not due to sadness at his grandmother's death alone, but to the shock of seeing his father as a vulnerable human being, as opposed to his idealized super-hero.

Mr. Miller's choice of friends also had a strong impact on his behavior. He had always considered himself to be an outsider, ostracized from most "in-groups" at school. He had difficulty finding an identity that suited him and became attracted to a group whose most salient characteristic was a strong emphasis on being a group of outsiders who did not identify with anyone else. Whereas Mr. Miller felt that other groups of people ignored or downplayed each other's troubles, he found that this group openly accepted his difficulties. However, from my perspective it seemed that they went beyond simply acknowledging difficulties, and instead tended to embellish and glorify personal problems. On the outset, it seemed contradictory that someone so averse to admitting the experience of emotion would be so engaged in a social group defined by the experience of painful emotion. However, this group served an important function in the maintenance of Mr. Miller's emotional avoidance. First, it played directly into his drive to escape his own problems by solving others', as the constantly melodramatic characteristic of this group of people provided a steady stream of crises on which to focus his attention. Even after he began to recognize the extent to which this behavior interfered with his ability to actually address his own issues, his continued association with this group sometimes made it difficult for him to make progress in addressing his own issues. Second, the group dynamic allowed him to act emotionally (usually with anger) without having to really feel his emotions. He could externally express himself in intellectualized, ruminative ways, as well as behaving in a number of ways that his companions encouraged, while not actually having to internally experience the real nature of his emotions. In this way, the group served a sort of compromise for him. He could vent his rising emotions in a way that did not threaten his narcissistic need to appear strong and in control.

After several sessions, Mr. Miller's acute distress faded, and his mood began to improve. His increased willingness to examine emotional experiences after they had occurred helped him learn to identify the different emotions he felt. As he became more able to identify accurately and describe his experiences, his comfort with them increased. This lead to a corresponding decrease in the distress he experienced by admitting the experience of emotion. He began to be less concerned about others' perceptions of his weakness due to having experienced emotion, which improved his day-to-day mood. He insinuated himself into the affairs of others less often, and began to reduce the embellishment and grandiosity of his day-to-day life. However, it is important to note that though he began to express a belief that the presence of emotion was not in and of itself evidence of weakness, he still maintained a high level of discomfort with the idea of actually experiencing them.

These changes were not without their own growing pains. Kohut (1977) and Winnicott (1965) have proposed that many narcissistic individuals experience an incongruence between their internal values or ambitions, and the way that they externally pursue those values. Some have suggested that boredom, which may lead to feelings of despair, is one of the possible results of such an incongruence (Svrakic, 1985; Wink & Donahue, 1997). This was born out in Mr. Miller's experiences as he made his changes. He had identified himself as the person who solved everyone's problems for so long, that the slow release of the "hero" identity left him in doubt as to who he really was. His reactions to this natural doubt and uncertainty of course included the occasional return to old habits. At these times, the motivations for these returns were discussed and an interesting motive appeared. Like his original ideas about the absence of distress being equivalent to positive emotion, the absence of crisis was equivalent to boredom. Mr. Miller believed that if there was nothing dramatic happening in the lives of his friends or family (and his own life by extension), there was nothing happening at all. This presented him with the incongruence between his internal ambition to protect people (primarily himself) and the external methods that he had used to do so. That is, Mr. Miller had a very hard time accepting that daily life did not necessarily entail dramatic events with potentially disastrous consequences, and the lack of excitement was so opposite to his internalized experience that it was often unbearable. His identity depended on the presence of a crisis to solve, and the absence of a crisis negated his assumed reason for being. A regular, day-to-day existence was boring, and boredom was equated with an unfulfilled, useless existence. Mr. Miller's earliest response to these calm periods was to seek out some problem to solve. In the beginning he did so more or less deliberately. He saw it as fighting boredom and stagnation, but frequent discussions about his choice of friends and places where he spent most of his free time were compelling enough evidence to help him rethink his pattern of behavior.

As Mr. Miller's mood and affect improved, and he began to be more stable on a day-to-day basis, he developed a very strong fear that some event would be negative enough that he would be unable to withstand its emotional consequences, and he would relapse into a depression similar to that which precipitated his suicide attempt. Mr. Miller had become aware for the first time of what it was like to be relatively happy, and he was simply terrified to lose that feeling. Despite the improvement in his mood and the gains he had made in therapy, his perception of his vulnerability did not diminish. Prior to beginning treatment, others were seen as tools with which to shield himself from distress and to promote his self-image. Now, he began to focus more intentionally on his own problems, and others became seen as obstacles that would stand in his way to addressing his own issues, and might damage or destroy his new-found happiness. Consequently, he began to display more overt signs of feeling vulnerable and fragile.

One session in particular served as a good example. He had been in therapy for approximately eighteen months, and his depression had been in remission for almost a year. As he identified the death of his grandmother as the point at which he had stopped being able to function well, the idea of the death of another loved one was particularly troubling. During this particular session, he revealed to me that a friend of his who had herself struggled with depression had taken a relatively large dose of an over-the-counter pain medication as a "pseudo-suicide attempt." Despite the fact that the majority of Mr. Miller's friends, including the young woman who carried out the act, considered this to be a cry for help and attention, he interpreted it as a legitimate attempt to commit suicide. He was convinced that should she have been successful at taking her life, he would have been entirely overwhelmed by grief and unable to function indefinitely. Mr. Miller's interaction with and response to his friend (who I will refer to as Ms. Smith) when he learned about her actions was as follows:

Mr. Miller: "I've heard you did something stupid the other night."

Ms. Smith: "Yes. I got real depressed, and decided to take a bunch of pills. I thought about killing myself, but it really wasn't serious."

Mr. Miller: "How could you do something like that? If you ever do anything like that again, I'll never speak to you again!"

When Mr. Miller related this to me, and I asked for his ideas about such a response, he responded that he knew that he "wouldn't be able to handle it if the worst happened. I just wanted to let her know how scared I was, and to distance myself from her so that if something did happen, it wouldn't hurt as much." As we began to examine the event in detail, it became increasingly clear that Mr. Miller's first concern was not for his friend's well-being, but his own. Though he acknowledged the difficult position in which she must have been, and despite the fact that he had been in similar circumstances, he was unable to empathize and respond in a way that expressed concern for her difficulty. Instead, he perceived that her action was a threat to his newly improved mental health.

Despite Mr. Miller's under-developed sense of self-efficacy, and his fears that distressing events would cause him an overwhelming amount of pain, he found that he had learned to withstand much of the pain he feared. One year into therapy, Mr. Miller learned that his other grandmother had developed a number of health problems that threatened her life. For several weeks, he was uncertain whether or not she would live, and questioned whether he would be able to withstand his grief. She lived for another year while undergoing chemotherapy treatment for cancer, but eventually stopped her chemotherapy and prepared to die. Mr. Miller spent three weeks uncertain of how he would react. During the funeral and weeks following, he continued to fight the tendency to suppress his emotions at home and around his friends and family. In therapy, he was much more willing to allow himself the experience of his grief. He also was able to discuss his feelings with his mother, which he had always been reluctant to do before. Through these experiences, Mr. Miller learned that he had more resilience than he had ever believed and showed a significant increase in the confidence he had in his ability to cope with difficult events.

One of the most gratifying improvements Mr. Miller made came after two years in treatment. Throughout therapy, his attitude toward me remained somewhat detached. As someone who often saw others as threatening, developing trust was something that was difficult for him. Though he never admitted to difficulty trusting me with anything specific, it seemed as though it took the majority of our time together for him to feel comfortable enough with me to become vulnerable in session. For him, there was perhaps a difference between the knowledge that my role as a therapist would prevent me from taking advantage of him or in some way breaking confidentiality, and the comfort that comes with believing that I only had his best interests at heart and would not judge him harshly. In exploring this, he realized that I bore some resemblance to many authority figures in his life, in that I played the role of someone with experience and expertise. He stated that it was very difficult for him to admit he needed therapy. He added that it was difficult for him to come to terms with the notion that he needed someone else's input on what was best for him, just as it was often difficult for him to accept that his parents could know better than he what was best for him. He was aware that there was a distinct difference between myself and other figures, such as his parents.

Throughout nearly three quarters of his time in therapy, Mr. Miller maintained an attitude of collegiality such as one might find between coworkers who only meet in the workplace. Though he grew to be able to discuss deeply personal things, they were always framed with a bit of emotional distance. Eventually however, he revealed he felt more comfortable hearing remarks he might perceive as criticism from me than from parents. This information indicated that in his transference experiences, he saw me in different roles at different points in his therapy—at one point, I was like a parent, and at other times I was like an equal. At times, he saw me as one who provided instruction, mentoring, guidance, and perhaps even a protective function that children often see in their parents. At other times, he related to me very much on the level of a colleague, or perhaps as a supportive friend, with whom he could share difficult information without the anticipation of a punitive or disparaging reaction. Also, he became able to grieve openly in front of me over his grandmother's death, and to tell me that he had been able to do the same with a few close family members. He relayed that, though it was still difficult, he did not see displays of emotion as weakness, if done in the right place and time. While he still maintained a sense that frequent display of emotion was a sign of weakness, his views of how weakness and emotion related to one another had shifted and now allowed him to process distressing events in a healthier way.

By this point in Mr. Miller's therapy, he had made great strides to address the issues that had given him so much trouble. He continued to struggle from time to time with his willingness to experience emotion and with his need to be in control of his emotions and reactions to things. He became much more comfortable with the notion that he changes and responds to events in the world, just as parts of the world change and respond to him, resulting in a dynamic relationship in which he is not always in total control. His experience in grieving for his grandmother showed him that his depressive emotions do not last forever, and gave him an increased sense of ability to manage them, leading to an increase in his sense of self-efficacy. Also, the frequency of his embellished stories decreased significantly, and he was much less likely to discuss things in abstract and intellectualized ways, instead being more able to make direct applications to himself. Though he continued to view others primarily in terms of the effect they might have on him and to be mildly suspicious of many, he also made great progress in being more trusting, genuine, and open with those to whom he was closest.

In contrast to these gains, he had much greater difficulty developing a stable sense of self-identity without the "hero" persona. A number of sessions were spent discussing the importance of this role and what it provided to him. For example, he was quite concerned whether any characteristics of the "hero," particularly the degree of care he professed to have for others, was really a part of his identity or if it was something he fabricated as part of the "hero" and now discarded once it was no longer useful. A review of his concerns and behaviors of the last several months since he had diligently begun to shed the "hero" showed him that he was indeed quite concerned about the welfare of those close to him. Therefore, he was able to accept that some of this persona was grounded in his true identity, and this served to ease some of his concerns and solidify his sense of self to some degree. While I remained uncertain about how much of his concern for others was out of legitimate interest in their well-being, or out of a need to protect himself, he showed genuine improvement in how he related and understood them.

COUNTERTRANSFERENCE

Much of the understanding of Mr. Miller I had was born out of the countertransference experiences that I had throughout the course of therapy. He was my first long-term patient, and the feelings I experienced during this time included excitement, interest (that approached amusement), boredom, frustration, and empowerment. Each of these gave me a bit more insight into his case, as I was able to use my reactions as ways to understand how others experienced him and the internal experiences he projected onto me. They also served to inform me of how my own experiences shaped the way that I would react to a narcissistic patient in ways that I could never have anticipated prior to working with Mr. Miller.

One of my earliest reactions to Mr. Miller's presentation was amusement. Often, his grandiose stories of fights, car races, drinking, and other activities seemed to be meant to convince me how tough and masculine he was. Consistent with many who have narcissistic conflicts, he acted as though he had something to prove to me—a need to show me how "together" he was in many aspects of his life. Part of what was interesting was the incongruence between his age/intellectual development and his boyish presentation. I often felt that he was trying to draw from me some type of approval or acknowledgment of how well he was able to perform these behaviors, and to establish either equality, or dominance with me. Despite his rather well developed intellect, he worked hard to impress upon me his ability and competence in a way that was reminiscent of a boy trying to demonstrate to his father or older brother that he could be independent and capable, while trying to win approval and acceptance at the same time. Due to this pull for a parental type of interaction, I realized to a better degree how little emotional nurturing he had experienced and how much he seemed to crave affirmation from a perceived parental/authority figure. At the same time, I remained conscious that in his narcissistic conflict it would be very difficult for him to recognize this craving, which therefore impressed upon me the amount of work we needed to accomplish.

I also realized that my amusement at his behavior and tendency to see him in a childlike light indicated a need of my own to be seen as a nurturing and caring person, much like a parent. It was important to me, not just as a therapist, but personally, that he come to trust me. I saw that this desire reflected a slightly idealistic belief I held about therapy—that all patients should like me and that I should be like a good parent. However, if I were not careful, I would begin to interact with and think of him as a child. Should he perceive me as treating him like this, his need to feel independent and competent could be challenged before he was ready and could damage the therapeutic alliance. It also could mean that I would reinforce his childlike sense of self and my need to be viewed as a kind, caring, parental figure.

Mr. Miller's crises also had an interesting effect on me. During the first phase of therapy, when they occurred on a weekly basis, it was quite easy for me to address them as patterns of behavior that allowed him to ignore his own problems by focusing on whatever outward event had taken place that week. I began to understand a little more deeply the value they had to him, as I found myself looking forward to hearing what he had engaged in each week. For my own part, discussions of them gave me some sense of satisfaction in that I felt I was finally getting to apply my years of classroom training to a real case, with a real person, who had real problems. I felt that my choice to become a clinician had been validated by the fact that I genuinely enjoyed working on a case that I knew was difficult, yet not overwhelming.

However, as he began to recognize the tendency of his crises to distract him from his emotions (and he began to regulate his reactions more effectively), there began to be lulls in the therapy where he reported very little from his daily life. These sessions were often slow, tedious, and boring. The fact was that his crises had made for easy subject matter, and even being able to point out this pattern was a relatively easy job. More difficult was the job of focusing therapy on the core issues of control and the loss of identity that he experienced with the reduction of the "hero" persona without these diversions. My frustration and boredom became a signal to me that he might be experiencing something similar. As he had given up a key component of his identity in the "hero," he was experiencing a significant degree of frustration as he struggled to understand who he really was and whether anything he had held onto in that persona was real. Also, as he experienced the lack of crisis in his life as boring, he projected an air of boredom into the sessions. In my interactions with him, I had become accustomed to frequent crises that could be exciting from a clinical standpoint. This absence of crisis was in some ways as dull for me as the therapist as it was for him as the patient, and we both became quite aware of the absence of excitement.

During these sessions, my mind would easily wander to other subjects. Sometimes I would miss something of importance that I only later recognized during supervision or examination of the video recording. As a way to compensate for these therapeutic missteps, I would begin to read more into some statements than may have been there, to make interpretations that were not as well founded as others, and to want to push his therapy faster than he was prepared for in order to feel that we were making progress again. As the week-to-week progress of therapy slowed, it was easy to consider terminating his treatment. After all, he had made progress, he was more stable, and his depression was in remission. However, when voicing these concerns to my various supervisors (of which I had three over the time I treated him), they often had similar responses to the effect that the most difficult work was still to come because we were now having to focus on his self-examination with fewer distractions. Up to this point he had been able to successfully defend the distress that would come with the deep and difficult examination of his core problems. Even as necessary as the first stages of therapy were, they were easier for him because they did not probe as deeply, and he was more aware of how much distress they were causing than he was of these more deeply seated issues. Had therapy been terminated at this point, he might have regressed into the same behavior that had led him to therapy in the first place and lost the progress of the previous months.

A particular supervisor remarked that the boredom or amusement I felt when listening to some of Mr. Miller's stories was likely indicative of the way others in his life experience their time with him. I was advised to use this by imagining how I would react if I were simply one of his friends or acquaintances as these reactions might then shed light on how he would interpret the actions and intentions of others. For instance, as I grew bored and disinterested with his stories, I imagined that as an acquaintance I might simply leave or stop interacting with him for a while, leaving him with a sense of abandonment. If I felt amused, I could see how others might try to manipulate him into fulfilling some other role, or treating him like a child, leaving him feeling resentful and angry. In those cases, I could better understand how he might feel ostracized or suspicious of others' motives, and how his need to prove himself might be reinforced in order to compensate for the conflicting feelings of weakness that accompanied a realization that others could affect him. I also learned that narcissistic individuals are likely to be charming and engaging at first, but as one gets to know them better, some of their traits will become tiresome and even grating.

An area in which I had some difficulty managing my responses in effective ways was in regard to Mr. Miller's intellectualization. As a student accustomed to discussions about abstract or theoretical ideas, it was easy for me to inadvertently accompany him into one of his intellectualized tangents about the nature of this emotion or that. When doing so, I would allow him to continue ignoring the personal impact of that emotion, and would inadvertently signal that it was acceptable for him to continue ignoring it. In fact, it took several sessions before I was able to recognize that I was doing this. Engaging in intellectualized discussion gave me a false impression of our progress; I would have the sense that we were doing therapeutic work while instead encouraging this tendency and actually holding back progress. In this way, I could easily understand how intellectualization made Mr. Miller feel better about things. He could use his more developed intellectual abilities to mask his underdeveloped emotional abilities, convincing himself that he was responding appropriately to his surroundings without realizing that he was stagnating his emotional growth. Also, I had a false sense of my own ability to conduct productive therapy. His need to feel able and competent in his experiences pulled for a similar reaction in me, in that my own needs to feel like a productive therapist were being met by this false sense of progress.

SUMMARY

Like many patients, Mr. Miller's course through therapy began with diagnosing and addressing a relatively obvious problem with depression, but his depression was quickly found to be influenced by a number of characterological problems. Many of his childhood experiences influenced these traits, including his parents' attitude toward the display of emotions, his and his father's respective physical disabilities, and the deaths of friends and family members. These experiences taught him that emotions were painful, damaging, and were to be avoided. Mr. Miller's narcissistic conflict was demonstrated by his frequent attempts to uphold a self-image of perfection that focused on being impervious to and controlling of emotion. He suppressed his emotions, and focused on solving the problems of others around him in order to avoid his own issues and to reaffirm his self-image. Additionally, he was likely to perceive even innocuous instances as personal threats, often acted impulsively and aggressively to these perceived threats, and spent considerable energy in therapy embellishing the details of these events in order to establish his image as a tragic hero. Other characterological issues Mr. Miller displayed were strong tendencies of splitting in his thinking, and weekly melodramatic crises.

Therapy lasted over two years and was successful in resolving his depression, and in addressing a number of his narcissistic tendencies. He became aware of his attempts to avoid facing his issues by focusing on others, of how the suppression of his emotions made it difficult for him to cope effectively with difficult events, and of his propensity to interpret things in extremes. His daily life became increasingly stable, and his ability to cope more effectively with distressing events improved significantly, as did his ability and willingness to recognize and experience a wide range of emotions. Despite many gains, he occasionally perceived threats where there were none, having difficulty forming trusting relationships. He also continued to be wary of emotional experience. Though his tendency to perceive them as inherently threatening was reduced, he remained uncomfortable with allowing himself to experience them.

My experience of Mr. Miller led to a wide range of my own feelings and reactions, including amusement, boredom, empowerment, and attachment. Each of these experiences served to give me increased insight into how others experience their time with Mr. Miller and how he might respond to them in turn, as well as a better understanding of his own experience as he projected many of his internal processes onto me during the therapeutic process. These experiences also taught me a great deal about how my own background and issues would affect my ability to conduct therapy, both in positive and negative ways.

NOTES

1. The author would like to express his appreciation for the supervision and guidance provided in this case: Dr. Norman Gordon & Dr. Tamara Penix.

2. Interestingly, Mr. Miller's mother never initiated a discussion of his case with me, and it was only necessary for me to discuss the case with her in order to try to corroborate some of his more incredible stories. She did not seem to need to know the details of his progress, outside whatever he discussed with her, and the need for her involvement was primarily on his side.

REFERENCES

Gabbard, G. O. (2003). *Psychodynamic Psychiatry in Clinical Practice*. Third edition. American Psychiatric Press, Inc., Washington, DC.

Kernberg, O. F. (1970). Factors in the psychoanalytic treatment of narcissistic personalities. *Journal of American Psychoanalytic Association*. 18, 51–85.

Kohut, H. (1977). *The restoration of the self*. New York: International University Press.

Kohut, H. (1997). *The restoration of the self*. New York: International Universities Press.

Svrakic, D. M. (1985) Emotional features of narcissistic personality disorder. *American Journal of Psychiatry*, 142, 720–24.

Wink, P. & Donahue, K. (1997). The relations between two types of narcissism and boredom. *Journal of Research in Personality*, 31, 136–40.

Wink. P. (1991). Two faces of narcissism. *Journal of Personality and Social Psychology*. 61, 590–97.

Winnicott, D. W. (1965). Ego distortions in terms of true and false self. In D. W. Winnicott, *The maturational processes and the facilitating environment* (pp. 146–52). London: Hogarth.

5

The Case of Mr. Schultz

Laszlo A. Erdodi[1]

CASE DESCRIPTION

Mr. Schultz was a fifty-year-old, unemployed single Caucasian male with a 4-year degree in liberal arts. He gave the impression of being an intelligent, articulate, highly verbal and well-read person. Decades before coming to our clinic, Mr. Schultz underwent therapy at another university counseling center for over a year. He described the experience as helpful and named it as one of the reasons for coming back. He was self-referred to the university's training clinic seeking help for low self-esteem caused by unresolved childhood traumas, conflicted relationship with parents, and an inability to keep jobs. In his past treatment over the course of two years, he cycled through several student therapists who tried a variety of approaches with him, including behavior therapy and acceptance and commitment therapy. With few exceptions, his symptom severity indices on a brief symptom assessment instrument routinely administered at the clinic were consistently below the clinical cutoffs. Nevertheless, he insisted on continuing to see his therapist, even requesting multiple sessions per week on occasions. He developed a reputation of being a challenging, long-term patient—a difficult case to conceptualize that elicited lasting countertransference feelings in his therapists.

At the time I contacted him over the phone to schedule an appointment, he had been on the waitlist for three months after his previous therapist had left the clinic when she finished her training. He expressed concerns about getting a male therapist, as he was promised and expected a female therapist. Finally, after some hesitation and reviewing his availability, he agreed to see me, and we set up an appointment for the same day. Half an hour before the scheduled time, he called in and cancelled the appointment.

When he finally came to the clinic a few days later, he appeared nervous and uncomfortable with the situation. He described his presenting problem as ongoing feelings of shame, self-doubt, and insecurity that had been haunting him since childhood. Mr. Schultz attributed this symptom cluster to the way his parents had been treating him. He grew up in a family environment where harsh, undeserved criticism, unpredictable anger outbursts, and generally cold, demeaning parenting were the norm. He used the metaphor of a "monkey on his back" to capture the nebulous set of negative emotions that he developed and that kept him from succeeding in several areas of life: school, career, romantic relationships. On the positive side, the way his core issue was symbolized indicated an indirectly expressed belief that the trauma history had not become an organic part of him. Rather, it was conceived as an external entity that, although attached itself to him and was parasitizing on him, had not become part of who he was. I interpreted this vivid expression of a mental separation between the self and pathology as a positive predictor of treatment outcome. Moreover, his ability to formulate a coherent narrative into the nature and origin of his psychopathology and his willingness to seek treatment for it was indicative of a high level of insight and motivation to change. The goal of therapy was clear: decrease the influence of this metaphorical monkey on Mr. Schultz's life. The path toward it turned out to be long and convoluted, with many turns and stops, and psychological sprinting and dragging of feet.

Initially, sessions were spent discussing his frustration with switching therapists, which centered on the fact that he had to start telling his life story all over again. He asked me if I had read his clinical records carefully, so that we could save time on his self-narrative. As he started sharing the narrative of his life with me, occasionally he paused and made a comment such as, "But I assume you already read about this" with a half smile on his face. Occasionally, he went as far as dropping off printed material for me to read at the front desk of the clinic between two sessions. These consisted mostly of printouts of his e-mail correspondence with important people in his life such as business partners, women he liked, and professionals. He wanted to check the appropriateness of his communication before (and sometimes after) he would actually send out the e-mail. Other times, he offered classic movies for me to watch to enhance my understanding of his complex case. He handed over the tape or DVD with a wide smile saying, "You'll enjoy this." He seemed oblivious to the boundary issues implicit in these gestures (i.e. him assigning homework for me) that were characteristic to the early stages of therapy. I understood his attempts to exert an inappropriate amount of control over the sessions and crossing the lines of socially defined roles as a compensatory mechanism meant to offset his anxiety and even out the perceived power imbalance between us.

During the first few sessions, Mr. Schultz told long, elaborate stories on topics seemingly unrelated to the presenting problem. These digressions took up most of the sessions, leaving little time to address the issues that brought him to therapy. He talked about current trends in macroeconomics, architecture, his interest in corporate decision-making, and a host of other highly abstract, neutral concepts. He seemed knowledgeable about topics and frequently used a didactic tone, asking me if I was familiar with something he was talking about or simply stating that I probably did not know what something meant. He then took the time to explain things to me and seemed to enjoy teaching me new things.

He also frequently mentioned his previous therapist, detailing how much she helped him understand himself in the context of his past. He spoke highly of her and repeatedly quoted a couple of interpretations she made about him, emphasizing how well they captured the essence of his condition, like "Your parents didn't want you to fail, yet they didn't want you to succeed either." I carefully monitored this tendency to idealize others in an effort to collect clinical observations to support my diagnostic conceptualization.

Following the initial period of ambivalence and awkwardness, however, the therapeutic relationship developed quickly and continued to improve throughout the time we worked together. The tangential stories were gradually waning, as more and more of later sessions were spent discussing clinically relevant, emotionally charged episodes from his far and recent past, and their implications on his life. After just a few sessions, Mr. Schultz became comfortable talking about his childhood traumas, current failures, and the discouraging prospects he was facing looking into the future: searching for a job without an ascending career path or even a solid work history or marketable skills, approaching retirement age with no savings, and trying to date interesting, "high quality" women without any impressive educational, occupational or financial achievements of his own.

Based on his clinical history, current presentation and pattern of symptom severity measured by a standardized rapid assessment instrument, he did not qualify for any major Axis I diagnosis. However, there was a consensus among student therapists and supervisors familiar with his case that he had an Axis II condition. He did not clearly match the DSM-IV criteria for a Narcissistic Personality Disorder (NPD), so I diagnosed him within the DSM-IV framework as Personality Disorder NOS with narcissistic features.

From a psychoanalytic perspective and in agreement with Gabbard (2000), I conceptualized Mr. Schultz as someone having prototypical narcissistic conflicts, falling somewhere in between the normal levels of narcissism that all people experience and a more severe form of NPD, characterized by a total lack of genuine interest in people and frequent, cold devaluation of others. He displayed some of the core traits that Akhtar and Thomson (1982) used to define NPD: he had unrealistic goals; he could not tolerate imperfection and desired admiration, although this last trait manifested itself in unusual ways. For instance, he liked telling stories that presented him in a favorable light, but at the same time he was reluctant to accept overt positive feedback from me. Following the more conceptual definition of pathological narcissism given by McWilliams (1994), Mr. Schultz fully fit the description: his identity and self-esteem was dependent on external validation, and his central conflict revolved around feelings of shame and self-doubt. To further refine his clinical profile, Wink's (1996) observation of narcissists also was relevant: he was chronically bored and dissatisfied with his work, and it was apparent that having a career served his need for self-affirmation rather than earning a living or following his intrinsic motivation in a given occupation.

As treatment progressed, and important details about his inner life were revealed, I incorporated multiple perspectives on NPD to build a case conceptualization of Mr. Schultz in an attempt to capture his complex presentation of symptoms. As the introductory chapter of this book delineates, the two most influential theorists of NPD, Kernberg and Kohut, agree that narcissism stems from an overcompensation for unmet needs during early development; however, their clinical conceptualization diverges at points, creating important differences in a treatment approach. I felt that a synthesis of their theories was needed to effectively address the complexity of my patient's psychopathology.

In accordance with Kernberg (1967), I believed that caregiver relations, chronic emotional deprivation, and repeated parental rejection were causal factors in Mr. Schultz's narcissism. His displayed grandiosity was an inaccurate, yet necessary, fantasy to retroactively compensate for these damaging early experiences. In his adult life this clinging to a desired, unrealistic self-image became a constant source of conflict and disappointment, and interfered with his interpersonal, occupational and emotional functioning. One of my treatment objectives was to gently, but systematically, confront and challenge this personality structure. I expected that a growing insight into the narcissistic compensatory mechanisms and their maladaptive nature would eventually produce clinically significant changes in his overall functioning.

I also relied on Kohut's (1968) approach to NPD, as I found it useful in conceptualizing several aspects of Mr. Schultz's presentation. The basic assumption remains the same: the lack of parental empathy during childhood contributes to a developmental arrest that later in adulthood manifests itself in narcissistic conflicts. Parents treat children as narcissistic extensions of themselves rather than autonomous individuals. Consequently, as adults, these children continue to rely on others for their excessive need for validation (Kohut, 1968). In addition to this narcissistic dynamic of the "looking glass self," Mr. Schultz's parents were constantly disappointed in their son and expressed their rejection in multiple ways through verbal abuse, withdrawing much needed emotional and material support, constant criticism, and neglect. Kohut (1968) postulated that some of the basic narcissistic conflicts are part of normal development—they only became dysfunctional if they went uncorrected, as the person was deprived of opportunities for healthy self-correction anchored in reality. I saw this as a major goal of therapy: to provide the patient with a chance to reexamine his reactions, assumptions and urges that were caused by early emotional deprivation and became the cause of his current pathology. Kohut (1968) advocates for a nurturing approach to treatment: instead of focusing on deconstructing and rebuilding a pathological personality structure in an inevitably confrontational manner, the therapist should provide some of the validation and support that the patient was lacking as a child.

Given the mixture of overt and covert narcissistic dynamics present in Mr. Schultz, I also tried to tailor my treatment to respond to this divergent symptomatology. Like many others, I believe that Kohut's (1984) sharp distinction between a confrontational and an empathic approach to narcissistic patients is a false dichotomy. Actually, I am convinced that alternating these two therapeutic styles was necessary for progress. I switched between the two approaches to adjust to the patient's presentation at any given time. During the early stage of therapy, I followed Kohut's approach, as I found it necessary for building a strong therapeutic relationship. As my alliance with the patient was strengthening, however, I gradually shifted to a Kernbergian style, starting to point out and challenge some of the patient's assumptions, desires, and interpretations. Although initially these confrontations were very subtle and often took several sessions to unfold, eventually the patient was able to tolerate and benefit from overt challenges to his ideas and statements.

Mr. Schultz fit Kohut's (1977) description of the prototypical narcissist in several aspects of his personality functioning: he displayed both defensive and compensatory structures, a general motivational deficit due to his preoccupation with unrealistic goals, and gave the impression of an idealistic adolescent whose thinking was not synchronized with the demands of real life. He called this symptom constellation *pseudovitality*: puerile enthusiasm that does not translate into mature productivity.

Kohut (1977) also provided criteria to evaluate the patient's readiness for termination. According to him, therapy could be considered complete when one of two goals has been completed. First, the primary structural deficit was exposed, processed and functionally restored. Second, the patient developed an understanding of and an ability to manage his emotional reactions that previously contributed to his core symptomatology. Although I found it difficult to unequivocally evaluate the degree to which either of these goals was fully achieved, I am confident in saying that Mr. Schultz made clinically significant progress towards both of them.

BACKGROUND INFORMATION

Mr. Schultz lived at the periphery of a Midwestern college town in government subsidized housing and had been chronically underemployed. He was the oldest of three sons and a daughter. During therapy, he shared very little information about his siblings. Instead, he focused on his parents while discussing his family. Growing up, his parents made sure to meet his basic material needs (food, shelter, clothes, health care), but otherwise he described the family environment as emotionally deprived at best, abusive at worst.

His early memories centered on the effects of a hostile family environment on his emotional development. He said he could only remember negative interactions with his parents. Regarding his father, he repeatedly stated: "I have no positive memories of my father. I have no negative memories of him either. He just simply wasn't there." This statement was contradicted by some of the anecdotes he told later in the therapy, which suggested that the father was a passive, yet unequivocally negative, influence in his life. Once he asked his father to teach him how to repair his car, which had broken down. He looked up, and said he would fix it himself later, as it was better not to involve his son— he would only slow him down. He also told his son not to touch the car, because he would likely make the problem worse.

This message of inadequacy was a recurring theme and penetrated the parent-child communication in Mr. Schultz's family. Through the years, this demeaning parental voice became internalized and became the "monkey on his back," his favorite image to describe his condition. This self-doubt had haunted him throughout his adult life. Interestingly, despite the pervasiveness of the trauma experience, he was able to detach himself from this sense of inadequacy and identify it as an acquired condition that could perhaps be deconstructed in therapy. Having preserved the duality of his sense of self and the developmental influences on him placed Mr. Schultz in a favorable position to change. He realized that his current self did not equal the sum of his experiences. Rather, he was an autonomous person who was determined to override some of the effects of his past.

Mr. Schultz described himself as a loner since he was a child. His early years were spent trying to escape the emotionally toxic home environment and spend as much time with his grandparents as he could. Inadvertently, he believed that these early experiences led him to becoming an introvert— a withdrawn child with an acquired "social startle reflex." He learned to be suspicious with people and anticipate hostile interactions. As a coping strategy, he adopted the "hit before you get hit" philosophy: when he became insecure in a social situation, he went on the offense by making sarcastic, mildly aggressive comments. Thus, even though he perpetuated a negative atmosphere around himself, he at least felt in control. I pointed out that, although this was a reasonable coping mechanism given the circumstances, as an adult the same strategy became counterproductive. He concurred, but this theme became dormant again for several more sessions until current life events brought it back to his focus.

Both of his parents had a significant history of trauma. As a child, his father witnessed the death of his father (Mr. Schultz's grandfather), allegedly while he was trying to save his son's (Mr. Schultz's father) life in a motor vehicle accident. Mr. Schultz had to reconstruct the story from hints divulged by other family members, as his father never talked about this to him—or anything else with emotional significance, as a matter of fact. I asked him if this incident and the secrecy in which it was wrapped helped him understand the father's personality, why he appeared to be a cold, withdrawn man who avoided contact with his children. Although he acknowledged the significance of the event, and paused for a moment, he did not seem to consider the hypothesis that his father's traumatic childhood could account for the dysfunctional behaviors that a generation later scarred him.

The patient's family history revealed that the maladaptive tendencies he described extended at least two generations back in time. His maternal grandparents were married because of an unwanted pregnancy—which is how his mother was born. Although the marriage was based on a dissonant relationship in which both of the spouses were unhappy (and her grandmother even contemplated a divorce), her physician advised her to stay married, given single women's financial fragility at the time. In Mr. Schultz's interpretation, his grandparents perceived his mother as the cause of the unfulfilled, erosive marriage.

Based on Mr. Schultz's description, his mother may have had some severe Axis II conditions herself. During his childhood, she was constantly jealous of her son because of the attention and affection he received from others, especially her parents. Likewise, she was generally unresponsive to her children. Even when she tried to show interest and affection towards her son, Mr. Schultz believed that she did so mostly to appear as a good parent to others, and did not seem to be aware of or concerned with the actual result of her actions. One time when Mr. Schultz was in the fifth grade, his mother brought a cake to school to celebrate his stage appearance in the class drama club. Although this seemed like a sign of affection, Mr. Schultz reported feeling very uncomfortable, wishing that he "simply wasn't there." This was partly because he was not used to his accomplishments being celebrated. But more to the heart of the matter, Mr. Schultz was bothered by how oblivious his mother to his discomfort over her actions and was actually taking pride in her public display of her motherly love at his expense.

A pervasive trauma of his early years, the mother's insensitivity remained unchanged well into Mr. Schultz's adulthood. Over the years, Mr. Schultz made repeated attempts to maintain at least a minimal contact with his mother, but was always met with rejection and demeaning remarks. She did not tolerate the slightest form of disagreement, a trait that made it virtually impossible for her son to establish any meaningful interactions with her. It struck me how, even in the face of mounting evidence that his mother was incapable of love or even being amicable toward her son, Mr. Schultz never gave up trying to create new opportunities to achieve a desired resolution.

His parents eventually divorced, and his father remarried. Regrettably, the stepmother essentially replaced his mother in the sense that she was equally rejecting. She was overtly and overly critical of her stepson, pointing out his perceived weaknesses as often as she had a chance. Moreover, she did everything she could to further widen the gap between him and his aging father. Despite the hopelessness he felt in this situation, Mr. Schultz tried to maintain at least a superficial relationship with his father. Once again, his efforts were largely unsuccessful and were further complicated by the increasing hostility of the stepmother, who exhibited paranoid delusions, and the progressing dementia of his father. When asked why he subjected himself to the perpetual humiliation and verbal abuse that came with his father's company, he said he was hoping that maybe one day things would turn around, and his father would finally accept him.

As therapy progressed, I was able to learn more about Mr. Schultz's childhood and adolescence. He spent his childhood wrestling with feelings of shame and rejection, while trying to discover who he really was. He coped with the emotional void created by his unresponsive parents by retreating to loneliness, where he felt safe. His favorite activities involved taking long walks in the woods, swimming in the lake by the grandparents' house, and developing hobbies that required social isolation, such as building model toys and snorkeling. It was apparent from his stories that he was not avoiding people per se. In fact, he craved the company of warm, accepting, inspiring adult figures. Yet his life situation led him to cope by escaping the noxious influence of his primary caretakers. Forced into loneliness by his circumstances, Mr. Schultz tried to make adaptive choices that would help him restore his emotional balance. Nature offered a convenient refuge for him during times of intense distress. However, his secessions were not always idyllic. The unmet needs for love and repressed resentment for ongoing emotional abuse sometimes surfaced in displaced aggression. For instance, his grandfather had an air gun and taught him how to use it. Subsequently, target shooting quickly became an obsession of his. He spent much time practicing, so that he became quite good at it. In his grandfather's backyard there were piles of organic waste that attracted little birds in search for food. Mr. Schultz would take out the gun, and shoot them down, one by one. He recalled feeling a strange satisfaction after shooting the foraging birds—innocent little beings feeding on human waste. As he was describing this, there was no sign of any sadistic gratification. On the contrary, he seemed disturbed by his own past behavior and was searching for a meaningful explanation. He interpreted the scene as a symbolic attempt to put an end to his own misery. "I was those little birds," he said: insignificant, fragile, trying to survive in a deprived, hostile environment and exposed to unpredictable victimization.

The motif of target shooting surfaced a few more times in the patient's self-narrative. One day his father took him to a state fair and became resentful when his son outperformed him in a target shooting game. Mr. Schultz described this event as being the way in which he came to have a "fear of success" throughout his early years. Even when he excelled at something, he was indirectly punished for it, as his success activated his father's insecurity, who responded by verbal degradation. Trapped in the impossible situation when both his achievements and failures elicited the same negative reaction from his parents who felt compelled to constantly criticize him, Mr. Schultz developed an ideation of grandeur in an attempt to rise above the situation.

His younger brother was facing similar pressures. At age nineteen, he committed suicide by hanging himself on a hickory tree in the backyard of the parental house. Even though the two siblings were fairly close as children, and he tried to protect the younger one from the negative parental influence as much as he could, Mr. Schultz only briefly mentioned the circumstances of his death. Later in therapy, he became tearful while talking about the tension and emotional void he experienced at home and asked: "What were my options? My brother couldn't take it any more, and he had his own way of ending it." My comments about his resilience and survivorship did not elicit any further response. His words dried up with his tears, and I wondered if this was the first time he had ever contemplated this possibility. He was similarly brief about his other brother, who severed his relationship with Mr. Schultz for reasons he did not discuss. He had not had any contact with him for over fifteen years.

After graduating from high school, Mr. Schultz went to college. Following his father's refusal to sign some documents that were needed for him to apply for financial aid, he had to finance his own education. And, despite having to work to support himself and pay for school, Mr. Schultz graduated on time with a degree in social sciences. He enjoyed the vibrant intellectual and social atmosphere of the college campus. He developed life-long interests in politics, anthropology, arts, economics, and sociology—all revolving around the concept of understanding human interactions at a systems level.

Years later he went to graduate school, but dropped out because of the difficulties he faced in a statistics class. He contemplated going back to finish his degree, but did not make any serious attempts to do so. He mentioned several times that he could go back any time he wanted, as he had the support of a professor friend. Yet, in looking at his ideas about graduate education, it seemed like the academia was more of a fantasy world, a narcissistic extension than a plausible avenue for achieving social status and gainful employment.

Mr. Schultz had a fractionated employment history: he frequently changed jobs, thus not giving himself a chance to build up a steadily developing career despite a wide range of interests and skills. He worked as a journalist, a salesman, and did a variety of unskilled manual labor that he did not like to discuss. For months, he kept retelling the same stories about why he left these jobs: he was bored, felt too good for the position, his boss was trying to cheat him, the restrictions imposed on him by the job hindered the expression of his creative force and interfered with his search for the truth. He often mentioned that he was due for a promotion in many of these positions, yet he still chose to leave.

His narratives were coherent, sensitive, and persuasive. Nevertheless, they did not sound very convincing to me. Given that he struggled financially and could not find steady work, it was hard for me to believe that he quit because of higher ambitions. It felt like there was more to the story, yet at the time it did not seem appropriate to challenge his explanations. Many sessions later, however, Mr. Schultz had a spontaneous revelation: "Maybe it wasn't boredom after all—maybe I was just scared of the responsibilities that would come with the promotion." Once again, he labeled this paradoxical feeling as "fear of success," showing some meaningful insight into his problems.

My impressions of him converged with this conceptualization: perhaps because he never experienced them as a child, strong positive regard felt strange to him. Not knowing how to respond to such positive feelings, he often just brushed them off, and escaped the situation. This created a perpetual state of dissatisfaction: he spent his life pendulating between a deep longing for acceptance and appreciation, but at the same time direct expression of admiration made him feel uncomfortable, as it was so foreign to him. At the beginning, his inability to take a compliment from me was paradoxical, given his diagnosis. It made me think that his narcissistic character distortion was incomplete: even though many of the grandiosity features were present, at the same time he was in touch with his vulnerabilities and was ready to talk about them openly. His awareness of his deficits was actually so strong that it prevented him from accepting genuine praise that he deserved. Ironically, this sensitivity to his shortcomings prevented him from indulging in healthy self-restoration by incorporating positive feedback into his self-image.

I also learned about Mr. Schultz's relationship history throughout the course of treatment. He explained that he started dating in college, but did not mention any long-term relationship from those years. Soon after graduating, he met an attractive young woman while volunteering at a social organization. She was the wife of a rich banker, intelligent, outgoing, and overall a glowing person. They quickly developed a mutual attraction. He greatly enjoyed her warm, supportive, affectionate personality—something that he always craved but never had. One day she invited him to her house, where the shared passion inevitably precipitated an outcome they both feared and wanted at the same time. Although Mr. Schultz expressed concerns that the husband might unexpectedly come home and shoot him, they ended up having sex in their conjugal bed. As the affair was slowly growing into a stronger bond, his insecurities bled through. He asked her why she was attracted to him, given that he was struggling financially, and her husband was a well-to-do businessman. She assured him that she did not care about money, and that she was in fact bored with her husband. Eventually, she left her husband for Mr. Schultz, and the couple moved to a different state. The following few months were perhaps the happiest period in his life. Enjoying the full benefits of a fresh start—with a new girlfriend and new job—he thrived in both major areas of life: work and love.

Of course, this idyllic state did not last very long. After initial successes as a photojournalist, he gradually became dissatisfied with the inherent limitations of his job. In his own words, he felt like a "big fish in a small pond." Although he quickly became popular among readers and respected among coworkers, Mr. Schultz wanted more: go beyond the reality framed by the simple values of rural America, uncover the complexity of life, and reveal some fundamental ambiguities embedded in the existence of a small, conservative community. Based on his description of these aspirations, they were thoughtful and indeed creative approaches to conventional topics. For example, instead of depicting the abundance of produce during harvest, as it was traditionally expected by the readership, he took pictures that focused on the untold story of seasonal workers, the forgotten force behind the richness of the fields.

Unfortunately, the editor was not responsive to his innovative vision. Although his productivity was appreciated, the community leaders were not comfortable with unorthodox ideas and styles. The editor made it clear to him that his work had to conform to certain guidelines, as the newspaper had an established profile and coverage that had to be preserved. There was some room for his creativity, but they did not consent to radical changes. Mr. Schultz interpreted this feedback as a rejection of his ideas and an attempt to stomp his talent. As a result, he became quickly disillusioned and contemplated leaving—the job, the town, the state.

In the meantime, the relationship with his girlfriend also became tense. She was bored and increasingly discontent with the rural lifestyle they were leading. She wanted to go back to school and applied to a graduate program of a prestigious university in their home state. Once she was accepted, the couple did not have any more reasons to stay, so they moved back to the college town where Mr. Schultz grew up. After the move, their relationship continued to deteriorate. She started becoming critical and demeaning toward him. "She turned into my mother," he said, during a dramatically insightful moment. A few months later, after a long agony, she decided to leave.

Mr. Schultz was hurt, but did not attempt to stop her. He concentrated his efforts on finding work and found a job in sales, and started earning a respectable income. His boss was very supportive and treated him like a son. Initially, he enjoyed the success. After a while, however, he felt a need for a change. When a friend invited him to California to look around and explore the job market there, he took advantage of the opportunity. He told his boss that he wanted to take a vacation and visit the West Coast. His reaction shocked Mr. Schultz: in a cold voice, he said that once he had used the same phrase himself, and never went back to his old job. Furthermore, he threatened Mr. Schultz that if this occurred, he would not pay his commissions that he still owed him. Betrayed by this surrogate father figure, Mr. Schultz went on the offense, and the boss settled the legal case amicably before it had a chance to go to the court. However, his ability to trust people who were close to him was once again compromised.

After that incident, his earning curve was gradually declining. He grew increasingly impatient and dissatisfied with sales jobs. He likened the industry to gambling: it took a large number of trials to finally succeed once. The local economy was also going through a recession, decreasing the overall volume of goods sold. Moreover, frequent rejections were a normal part of salesmanship, but extremely difficult for him to handle. Although logically he understood that the profession was a numbers game, and being turned down all the time was inherent in the nature of the job, it was still too threatening for him to constantly experience it. For all these reasons, Mr. Schultz decided to quit looking for new work after his last sales job ended, and he was laid off. He lived off of his slim savings, and after it ran out, he relied on need-based financial assistance from the government. Occasionally, he took small, unskilled jobs like landscaping and painting houses to complement his income, but he was ashamed of those, and refused to even consider pursuing any of those venues to earn a steady income. He thought of manual labor as an insult to his superior abilities. Interestingly, he did not mind raking leaves and painting barns as a volunteer for the local church or nonprofit organizations that he liked and supported. However, he dreaded the idea of being identified with a blue-collar, low-prestige profession. Instead, he preferred staying home, reading books, watching educational programs on TV, and socializing with highly educated people, while barely surviving on his welfare check.

Shortly thereafter, Mr. Schultz had one long-term romantic relationship with a nurse that lasted four years. He described her as quiet, loyal, and meek, yet also withdrawn and simple-minded. He could not say anything negative about her except for the fact that she was unable to fully capture his interest. The fact that he had difficulty engaging her in intellectually stimulating conversations became a growing source of frustration that eventually led to the break-up. Mr. Schultz seemed to have been attracted to highly intelligent and accomplished women, and became easily bored with anyone less than that.

TREATMENT HISTORY

As he first walked in the therapy room, Mr. Schultz was visibly anxious and uncomfortable with the situation. He expressed his doubts about my ability to help him, given that I was a new male therapist unfamiliar with his case. I tried to validate his feelings by acknowledging that it took a fair amount of trust for someone to feel comfortable with that risk. While fighting my own countertransference feelings as a reaction to his subtly devaluing statements, I was sincerely hoping to earn enough of his trust to engage in a therapeutic interaction from which he would benefit. During our first session he named two main objectives for treatment: to improve self-esteem by eliminating feelings of insecurities and self-doubt, as well as to obtain and maintain a job. Both of these were challenging in different ways for him. But, shortly after we started working on these goals, I learned that they were essentially one complex task: working toward him feeling comfortable enough with himself that he could adjust his expectations and realize his potential in more realistic terms.

The next several sessions appeared initially to be off-track from his stated goals: Mr. Schultz carefully avoided any topic that was remotely related to his stated goals in therapy. He gave long, tangential speeches on safe, neutral topics. He spent more time checking my general knowledge on macroeconomics and cinematography than talking about why he was there.

Looking back, I realize that it was my turn to learn at that point: being trained in the time-limited tradition of the empirically supported treatments, I could not help keeping an eye not only on the clock, but also on the calendar. I felt that Mr. Schultz was making no progress whatsoever after four or five sessions, and the thought of that made me feel uneasy. At the same time, I was sensing that it would be both counterproductive and impossible to attempt to speed up the process. Therefore, a major function of the clinical supervision became learning to accept the slower rate of progress stemming from a different clinical presentation. I had to fight my own doubts and rescale my expectations in a very similar way that I expected my patient to do. These parallel processes were both heuristic and cathartic. They provided clarity and an experiential basis for my clinical work at the same time. As I slowly developed a more intimate understanding of the nature of the patient's conflict, I could build a model of his emotional functioning using my own countertransference as raw material.

As I was wrestling with these intellectual and emotional tasks, the therapeutic alliance was improving quickly. Beginning the second session, Mr. Schultz started giving me a synopsis of his life. His narrative was coherent, well formulated and presented in a chronological order. He told the story of his life in a matter-of-fact, Hemingway-like style, with little interpretation, and even less emotion. However, he was gradually growing comfortable with delving into the emotional core of his trauma history. Similarly, at the beginning, he seemed a little annoyed that he had to repeat the story of his life once again because of switching to a new therapist, but with time he stopped mentioning it. In many ways, I felt that he was testing me out to see if I would respond much like the many other men in his life who had rejected him.

The next several sessions led to an increased therapeutic alliance and a series of changes. The proportion of time spent talking about tangential topics gradually decreased. More sessions were spent discussing issues that were relevant to his presenting problem. Also, he made fewer references to his previous therapist. Similarly, he engaged in fewer didactic episodes when he was trying to teach me about something that randomly came up during our discussion. Overall, his narcissistic defenses were weakening. I was very pleased to see this for two reasons. First, it made it easier for me to work with him. Second, and more importantly, I felt like we had a chance to work on the issues that brought him in therapy in the first place. Although fifteen sessions had transpired, my expectations about the nature and pace of progress changed. I was developing insight into the nature of the narcissistic conflict as I began to understand and accept that change would happen slowly. Also, I learned to appreciate small signs of progress, and point them out to the patient when appropriate so that we could build upon them.

As therapy continued, Mr. Schultz shared layers of his personality that were getting closer to the core. Despite his maladaptive, narcissistically driven tendencies, he managed to create and maintain strong, meaningful friendships that spanned over decades. He took pride in some of his high profile friends: university professors, computer programmers, lawyers, architects, and automotive engineers. He liked to describe their accomplishments and indulge in "glamour by association." It was interesting to see how Mr. Schultz solved some of the narcissistic conflicts inherent in these friendships. These prototypically successful people seemed to serve as a narcissistic extension of himself and, as such, enhance his image. His face lit up while telling stories of riding with a friend in a convertible sports car in downtown Chicago, or when a prestigious architect firm wanted to hire him without any relevant professional experience as a result of a friend's recommendation.

In contrast to the needs met by these friendships, Mr. Schultz felt worse about himself when he compared himself to them. He attenuated this threat by focusing on how much the lives of these people were consumed by their careers and the inevitable regrets that successful people have looking back in life. This gave him an opportunity to describe the benefits of his lack of commitment to any single life goal. At the same time, he realized that the lack of pressure to persevere (not having to pay mortgage, take care of a child, no tenure track position) contributed to his lack of long-term vision and caused him to be trapped in short-term pursuits that never accumulated to a larger material or emotional investment in something—a house, a job, a person, an idea. His basic needs were always met to some extent (working temporary menial jobs that "paid the bills," brief encounters with women, joining social organizations), so he lacked a strong incentive to push himself and follow some of his numerous ambitions (becoming an architect, college professor, rich businessman) that over the course of his life became reduced to escapist fantasies.

This strange duality defined Mr. Schultz. As treatment unfolded, I noticed that episodes of realistic, but depressive, self-reflections were alternating with narcissistic ideations. Some days he came in depressed, and gave me a realistically-based synopsis of his life and his accomplishments (or the lack thereof). During these times, he had amazingly clear insight into the nature of his problems. He admitted to mistakes he had made in life, and how his choices contributed to his current situation. Inadvertently, these stories had a tendency to get caught in a downward spiral of depression, and it was clear that his dysphoria was not offset by realistic feelings about his abilities to reach important goals. In these times, childhood traumas were evoked, retold, and tears were shed. He shared some of his most intimate stories with me that helped me understand the history and quality of his emotional experiences.

Mr. Schultz's clinical presentation was consistent with Wink's (1991) studies on narcissism. He described two subtypes: the Grandiose-Exhibitionist and the Vulnerable-Sensitive. Although both types shared common features (self-indulgent, impulsive, controlling, intolerant and demanding), there were also important differences between them. The former was described as sociable, self-centered, exploitive, assertive, arrogant, attention seeking, but unfulfilled and pessimistic. The latter was described by the following traits: vulnerable, worrisome, emotional, defensive and tense. Interestingly, Mr. Schultz had qualities of both types. At times, he behaved as a prototypical overt narcissist: he told stories about his past grandeur, others' admiration of him, and the special treatment he deserved and received from others. During these periods he was prone to violate the patient-therapist boundaries by making inappropriate jokes, trying to extend the conversation beyond our clinical work, and making demeaning comments about me. He seemed genuinely oblivious to these violations of the therapeutic framework. Other times, entire sessions passed without projected grandiosity and devaluation (which masked feelings of insecurity) surfacing. Rather, he presented himself as a depressed man who was tragically aware of his own limitations and was committed to working through his expressed feelings of inferiority. It was fascinating to see the two faces of narcissism in the same person: the self-constructed image of a confident, successful man that metamorphosed into a more sensible, hurting person very much attuned to his vulnerabilities. Experiencing this duality was like watching a running engine made of transparent material: one could see the mechanism by which the pistons and valves worked together to transform one form of energy into another.

Although enlightening and a valuable training experience, these divergent self-presentations were difficult to handle from a treatment perspective. Clinically, Mr. Schultz was a different person depending on which of these subtypes presented themselves during any given session. I found that when Mr. Schultz displayed overt, classical narcissistic tendencies, little progress was made. Often, the session involved him talking to me without expecting or being receptive to any feedback. On days like this, he had a self-assured smile on his face and was telling me about his ambitious ideas, plans, and past accomplishments. These stories were peppered with anecdotes in which he was the dominant figure, a confident man who made things happen: how he found a girlfriend for his best friend, how he seduced the beautiful wife of a rich banker, how he impressed his girlfriend's friends at a party by taking over the discussion and entertaining them, and how he, as the most talented of the journalists, was assigned to interview the lieutenant governor visiting the small town. This 'overt narcissist mode' was marked by distinctive affect. His face would light up, he laughed, and visibly enjoyed re-creating the narrative. Through the course of treatment, I learned to recognize this specific affective display as the manifesto of an activated narcissistic conflict. If he could not obtain his father's approval so necessary for a boy's developing self-image, he went on the offense symbolically defeating the oppressive paternal figure, taking pride of this symbolic victory. Conversely, when the covert cluster was dominant, he felt comfortable disclosing his vulnerabilities, responded to my comments, and was developing insight into his patterns of thinking, feeling and acting. Similarly, this modality of his personality functioning was accompanied by a characteristic affect. He was quiet, paused frequently, waited for my response, seemed consumed by melancholy and even became teary on occasion.

Once I realized how discrepant the sessions were as a function of his presentation, particularly how evasive he was toward self-exploration while in a more overt orientation, I started responding to him differently. Specifically, I tried confronting his overt narcissism and challenging his exaggerated statements. Despite some partial success in addressing his overzealous, fantasy-dominated rhetoric, I was unable to facilitate his transition to a more realistically-mediated middle ground, where meaningful therapeutic interaction could happen. I slowly learned that challenging the overt narcissist was largely ineffective, and I was left to wait until he came to session with a more covert presentation. I also tried to engage him in a way that the content and themes of our session would extend beyond our fifty minutes together and last until I would meet him the next week. Therefore, I asked him difficult questions on topics important to him and reminded him to ponder them during the following week before he left, in a hope that his imagination would be captured by actual problems, and he would be working on realistic solutions instead of engaging in escapist fantasy.

Despite my best efforts to stabilize this changing symptom presentation, and prolong the mindset in which therapy could progress, he continued to switch between these two sides without any predictable pattern. For example, after he identified unemployment as the core problem, we explored possible jobs he might be qualified and willing to do. I asked him to make a list with the types of work he could see himself doing, and bring it to the next session. However, the next time I saw him he came in with a new plan: he wanted to start his own web design company. A year later, this business had not generated any revenue, but at times he still enjoyed the idea of being the founder, owner, and CEO of a start-up company that grew out of a bold idea, defying the skepticism of businessmen and professionals who were presented with the concept.

Although I learned to view this alternation in his affect and cognition as an organic part of his diagnosis, at some level it still continues to perplex me how split his self-representations were and how these two conflicted sides of Mr. Schultz were oblivious to one another. When depressed, he openly acknowledged the nagging self-doubt, shame, and insecurity that inhibited him from being proactive, productive and happy. He also pointed out several of his counter-productive strategies that were used to cope with his low self-esteem. He was aware of his social skills deficits, and he was willing to work on correcting them. However, when the other Mr. Schultz walked into the therapy room, I was facing a very different patient: someone who was confident, assertive, and not very open to change—someone who enumerated his many different strengths, past successes, and future potential. This patient did not want a therapist—he wanted an audience. Perhaps his damaged self-image resulting from chronic deprivation of attention from significant others demanded a belated compensation. Nevertheless, this kind of ego gratification was not facilitating his adaptive functioning on the long run.

Mr. Schultz produced detailed and coherent narratives that helped me reconstruct the psychological ontogeny of his problems. Many of his accounts were emotionally intense and provided me with good examples of what kind of experiences shaped his personality as he was growing up. They sounded authentic, as they seemed to recreate the affective state the original events produced in Mr. Schultz decades ago. However, after having heard many of these anecdotes, I noticed that they started repeating themselves. Also, the cathartic component was often missing. Reliving the trauma through story telling did not relieve the pain they elicited. On the contrary, they seemed to preserve the suffering by encapsulating them into well-polished narratives.

As treatment progressed, he slowly abandoned telling stories from the past as prompts for self-exploration. Eventually, there was no need for a background narrative for Mr. Schultz to focus on the immediate issues he was wrestling with. Finally, after a year of therapy, we could have a session that focused entirely on intense, painful conflicts, involving some of his deepest fears and regrets, without the break provided by anecdotes. He reached a point where he talked openly about his transference feelings, how he was worried that he would disappoint me, and his shame and rejection felt in response to my perceived (and sometimes real) frustration with his progress. In return, I started using our therapeutic relationship and the evolution of the dynamic between us as a model to understand his interactions with others. We reached a stage where we both felt safe discussing negative emotions (frustration, impatience, discomfort) elicited by each other openly, without defenses and without fearing negative reactions from the other. Moreover, we could use those self-reflections therapeutically, to process the past and adjust the future. At that point, I had the strange feeling that I vicariously underwent a therapeutic change myself: along with Mr. Schultz, I learned how to handle sensitive, intensive emotions in a safe and clinically productive manner.

I would like to believe that the way our relationship changed during the course of the therapy was symbolic of not only his trauma history, but also his capability to make adaptive changes. Initially, he likely perceived me as another authority figure who would criticize and reject him. Thus, his defenses were activated frequently during this early stage of therapy. With time, he slowly learned to trust me. He saw that I was a stable, reliable object who was there for him and genuinely tried to help. There was a tipping point (or more like an abrupt change in slope on the imaginary graph of the development of our therapeutic alliance) where his grandiosity and self-righteousness almost completely disappeared in sessions. I could not tie this important development in our therapeutic interaction to any specific event, but I interpreted it as evidence that he no longer felt the need to retreat in his fantasy life or go on the offense to feel safe. Instead of meeting his needs in maladaptive ways, he decided to confront his fears and insecurities: he abandoned the narcissistic defenses and made the difficult choice of replacing them with mature strategies. He started accepting some of his irreversible deficits (lack of career, family, wealth) and refocusing on synchronizing his existing potential with more realistic expectations. During this process, I developed an appreciation for long-term psychotherapy. My work with Mr. Schultz made me understand how and why treating Axis II pathology could only be done with much patience and over a long period of time. The adaptive shift in attitude, cognition and emotional self-regulation described above occurred slowly, in small steps. I believe that the additive effect of these incremental changes is a core feature of treating NPD. In many ways, psychotherapy is meant to help the patient better adjust to life in general, recognize its patterns, its short and long cycles, and how the individual contributes to some of the outcomes. Essentially, the temporal dimension must be modeled in therapy to establish a larger context in which the patient can experience how his choices are reflected in events around him. This is difficult to do in a few, highly structured sessions. It takes time for psychopathology to unfold in front of the eyes of the therapist in its full richness. This process is crucial for therapeutic change, and cannot be accelerated by imposing deadlines and structure.

COUNTERTRANSFERENCE

One of the major obstacles that I had to overcome in the course of treating Mr. Schultz was my reluctance to trust my own intuition regarding his core psychopathology. After all, a clinical case conceptualization of narcissistic pathology requires careful monitoring and interpretation of intrasubjective events that are not available to external observers. Being trained in an empirical tradition, the automatic reaction I had to my own introspection was skepticism and discomfort. As part of my training in treating Axis II psychopathology, I had to absorb and internalize Kohut's (1987) axiom that a therapist must "assume that our understanding of what is going on in the patient will help us to make him more mature, more adapt." In other words, engaging the patient in a therapeutic dialogue, listening to him and reflecting his thoughts back to him facilitates an adaptive restructuring of his personality. I had to learn to take reasonable risks in my case conceptualization, and be comfortable following my clinical intuition.

The other major task was recognizing and processing my emotional reactions to the patient, which were particularly strong in the earliest sessions. Although historically countertransference has been viewed negatively, as a distortion that a therapist makes about a patient, more balanced interpretations have been recently introduced into the psychoanalytic literature. Eagle

(2000) summarized the research on countertransference by suggesting that it could be interpreted as a reflection on either the analyst's or the patient's emotional functioning (or both). His summary is based on earlier ideas by Racker (1968), who pointed out that the therapist was in the unique position of being the interpreter of the patient's unconscious processes, but at the same time being affected by them. Therefore, the accuracy of the clinical interpretation and the clinician's reaction to the patient are dependent on each other, making it an imperative for the therapist to closely monitor his countertransference. Jacobs (1991) gave a detailed example of how the analyst and the patient are yoked together by the similarity of their past conflicts, the only important difference being that the former has developed an awareness of them and has learned how to manage them effectively, while the latter is controlled by them in the present. Racker (1968) acknowledged and emphasized the ambivalence of countertransference feelings in the therapeutic process: they can impair or enlighten the clinical judgment, depending on how they are managed.

Experiences of countertransference started instantly, as the patient's self-doubt and ambivalence about restarting therapy were projected onto me. He openly voiced his skepticism about my ability to help him, yet he agreed to "give it a try." Although I expected this kind of dynamic to develop between us, and I thought I was mentally prepared for this, it did affect me in a number of ways.

First, it elicited a generalized negative emotionality, which could be best described as a combination of resentment (having to deal with an oppositional, resistant patient), frustration (perceived inability to make therapeutic progress), anger (emotional reaction to subtle forms of aggression) and insecurity (emerging doubts about my skills as a therapist—perhaps the core emotion in my countertransference). Although I had developed a basic sense of clinical competence by that time, it was very difficult for me not to take Mr. Schultz's comments personally or further, to recognize them for what they were: opportunities to understand the inner mechanisms of his emotional functioning. Even though I made conscious efforts to label my countertransference and process those feelings in the appropriate context, initially I could not fully appreciate the chance to vicariously experience life, people, and interactions the way Mr. Schultz did. Without realizing what he was doing, he allowed me to sample the gamut of emotions he was wrestling with himself. Without realizing what I was doing, my initial reaction to him was similar to that of most other people in his life: irritation and rejection. I felt his pain immediately, but at the beginning I did not know how to manage it in a way that would be therapeutic for the patient and bearable for me. It took many hours of clinical supervision from a therapist with vast experience in Axis II psychopathology, reading articles on narcissistic conflicts, and personal reflections on my interactions with this patient until I could finally capitalize on my countertransference feelings rather than letting them interfere with my clinical work. Understanding their function was key for me: that is, they were markers of a maladaptive interpersonal dynamic that could be explored and capitalized on throughout treatment. The turning point in this process was realizing that countertransference was (or could be made into) an opportunity, not an obstacle.

Second, at the beginning, my poorly managed countertransference interfered with my performance as a therapist. Too much of my mental energy was absorbed by ongoing attempts to control my emotional reactions to the patient. As a result, I was not as clinically effective as I expected myself to be. Of course, these deficiencies only became obvious to me in retrospect. At the time I was so focused on making it through the given therapy session, that I became oblivious to certain clinically relevant behaviors. Specifically, on occasion I failed to ask appropriate and necessary follow-up questions. As a result, I missed opportunities to explore a potentially important conflict when the patient created a context for it through hints and ambiguous statements, and it would have been natural to inquire about them. I would like to think that most of these missed clinical data were obtained later, as there was significant redundancy in Mr. Schultz's self-narratives, but I have no way to be certain of that.

Finally, Mr. Schultz's transference had a demoralizing effect on me. Although it was my decision to take on a complex clinical case with Axis II psychopathology, after the first few sessions I started to develop certain doubts. I noticed that I was becoming tense before sessions and exhausted afterwards—a lot more so than I did with any other clinical case, and in qualitatively different ways. For the first time in my clinical training, the interaction with a patient was aversive. Albeit briefly, I started questioning myself regarding my clinical skills, personal aptitude, and even career choices. The lowest point of my manifest countertransference was a sarcastic comment I made about my patient during group supervision when a colleague asked me why Mr. Schultz came to therapy. Caustically, I replied that most likely because nobody else would listen to him for fifty minutes for the amount of money he paid for the session.

Soon after uttering that, I realized I was getting trapped in the same web of negative emotions Mr. Schultz was struggling with. Moreover, it also became clear that until I found a way to effectively manage my countertransference, I would not be able to help him progress toward his goal. It was my turn to develop some important insights. Instead of removing the monkey on his back, I developed a smaller one on my own. This recognition emphasized my need and precipitated my efforts to reevaluate my countertransference in a clinically productive way. I perceived it as a twisted form of experiential learning: it gave me a taste of what it might feel like to *be* Mr. Schultz—develop negative impulses (and occasionally acting on them) in the face of mounting frustration, despite the fact that they were only making relating to others even more difficult. Like a natural experiment, my countertransference allowed me to model the dynamic between Mr. Schultz and the significant objects in his life.

When I decided to take up Mr. Schultz as a patient, I thought I was mentally prepared for the unique challenges that Axis II psychopathology brought into the therapy room. Nevertheless, the initial contact was more stressful than I anticipated. The patient activated certain negative emotions in me that I had only heard about before from therapists who routinely treated patients with personality disorders. It was not the typical "performance anxiety" that a new patient commonly elicits in a new therapist; it was not the helplessness felt when faced with a complex clinical case that had no clear solution. It was not the repulsion that one might feel trying to treat antisocial personality disorder or a child molester. He elicited feelings of incompetence in me as a therapist, from a caustic comment about my lack of knowledge of the clinic's computer system when I had difficulty printing his receipt ("I'll let you guys figure out how your computer works") to a global evaluation of my lack of clinical skills ("I'm not sure that you can help me").

Looking back, these comments have a different meaning for me. Now I fully understand that they were not a deliberate character attack, but a desperate attempt for Mr. Schultz to preserve a sense of control over a stressful situation. He came to me for help resolving his lifetime conflicts, but he did not yet feel comfortable sharing his story with me. Therapy made him once again feel vulnerable, and he only knew one way to manage the feeling: by going on offense. There is an important difference between knowing and feeling, though. The mere awareness of the psychological function a behavior has does not necessarily eliminate the visceral reactions it elicits. Nevertheless, it makes it easier to process in constructive ways. I still had to experience countertransference, and wrestle with it from session to session, until I could profit from it instead of being encumbered. I found the experiential component to be of utmost importance, and I think that no amount of reading can substitute for the heuristic value of going through it.

Supervision from a psychoanalytically oriented faculty experienced in treating Axis II patients greatly facilitated my process of moving beyond this difficult start while building rapport with the patient and preserving morale. Had I not prepared for it, I would have been confused and discouraged by countertransference. During supervision meetings, however, I was reassured that this was a normative stage in establishing therapeutic alliance. Of course, this awareness did not completely eliminate the negative feelings, but at least it transformed anxiety, boredom and frustration into a nervous, yet hopeful, expectation of a meaningful continuation. Understanding the nature of the countertransference I was experiencing, and that this was a natural component of therapy with this population, helped alleviate most of its negative effect. Moreover, instead of perceiving it as an obstacle, I was encouraged to explore it in search for therapeutically enlightening discoveries.

Following this guidance accomplished two goals. First, it helped me manage my insecurities by interpreting them in the context of my patient's complexities: labeling them as countertransference and identifying their functions, both in the patient and in myself. Second, analyzing my reactions to the patient's behavior led to a better understanding of the dynamics of his personality. *Experiencing* what it felt like to interact with him during an episode of narcissistic rage provided invaluable clinical data above and beyond his self-constructed narrative. Of course, the former (managing countertransference) was the prerequisite for the latter (benefiting from it): it would have been impossible for me to draw valid clinical inferences while under the influence of the strong emotional reactions elicited at times by the patient.

Fortunately, my intensely uncomfortable initial reactions dissipated quickly. They downshifted to impatience and frustration with lack of progress, and eventually metamorphosed into feelings of empathy and even admiration at times. Looking back, I am glad it happened. First of all, by now it became my personal, inner marker of potential Axis II pathology. Next time when I interact with a patient who elicits similar feelings, it will prompt me to assess for a potential personality disorder. Second, it provided me with an in vivo simulation (sometimes too vivid for comfort, perhaps) of what other people must have felt like while interacting with Mr. Schultz. For the first time I understood the true meaning of the doctrine that therapy is a sample of the patient's general functioning: it can be used to extrapolate how he would behave outside of the therapy room—and in this case, what kind of reaction he is likely to generate in others. Finally, it provided me with exposure to a situation that threatened my sense of competence as a developing clinician. Facing it, resolving it, and turning it around into a learning opportunity was a challenge routinely faced by therapists, but I had not experienced that myself. This case was my initiation to a fascinating population of patients that is nevertheless difficult to work with at times. I learned to see countertransference as a unique opportunity to understand the patient rather than an "occupational hazard." For all these reasons, I am grateful that I met Mr. Schultz. In a strange way, he taught me at least as much about psychotherapy as I taught him about himself.

SUMMARY

Mr. Schultz came to see me initially to continue his journey toward self-discovery. A strange mix of eagerness and avoidance, he was reliable in attending sessions and unpredictable in his therapeutic progress. He wanted to break away from his traumatic past that he identified as the main source of his misfortunes. At the conclusion of our work together, he made a few important realizations. First, despite the gravity of the old traumas, his past does not have a deterministic relationship with his future: there is room for change, healing and growth. Second, he is an active agent in shaping his life: what he does in the present influences his opportunities in the future. He is both a victim of and a contributor to his misfortunes. Third, certain injuries that he has suffered and choices that he has made have immutable consequences, and the best way to manage them is to accept them, and learn how to live well despite the losses.

These insights translated into significant improvements in several areas of his life. He became less vulnerable to depression: negative life events no longer spiraled into a paralyzing episode of self-doubt and guilt. His interpersonal functioning was similarly enhanced by the ability to take another's perspective, and conceptualize relationships as a dynamic exchange instead of a social game that revolved around him—with all the glorious and humiliating consequences of that fantasy. Finally, he became more adept at recognizing and processing his emotions. His presentation during sessions was becoming increasingly more stable, balanced, with fewer eccentricities.

Other aspects of his functioning remained unchanged. At the time of termination, he was still unemployed, living off of fantasies of financial success and social prestige, while generating creative excuses why he would not consider investing time and effort in a feasible, yet modest career choice. Nevertheless, towards the end of our work together, my insistence on confronting him with his rationalizing tendencies produced one important (although of questionable utility) change in his self-conceptualization: he started to view his behavior as partly a result of his personal choice as opposed to strictly a linear transformation of childhood maltreatment. I would like to think that he left therapy equipped with the tools to transform this realization into a more fulfilling existence.

I believe that our therapeutic alliance was the central element of our work together. I learned how consuming it could be to do therapy with patients whose psychopathology is an organic part of their personality structure. It was an intense experience that definitely tested the limits of my clinical competence. It also modeled for me that real change and growth can only occur if one is willing to expose and embrace his vulnerabilities in constructive way. In this sense, I am noticing remarkable parallel processes: Mr. Schultz walked into the therapy room filled with doubt, pain, a chronic sense of dissatisfaction with life and suspicion towards me. I greeted him with some anxiety and the anticipation of a complicated, conflictual clinical case. After the year and a half we spent together, we both changed. The insecurities metamorphosed into understanding, acceptance, and the humble confidence of the person who did not solve his issues, but came to terms with his limitations.

At the end of our first session, as Mr. Schultz was getting ready to leave after a tense, unpleasant fifty minutes, I automatically went to shake his hand. He pulled back, and with a nervous laughter he told me that he would rather not, as a handshake had unpleasant connotations for him—the end of an interaction, which seemed a premature, hence inappropriate gesture at the time. At the end of our last session, he initiated a handshake. I reminded him of our interrupted ritual from over a year prior. It was the first and last time we shook hands. He wished me well, and predicted a successful clinical career for me. His words were wrapped in a calm half-smile. I felt that we finally came full circle. He left without looking back. I returned to my desk with a strange, uplifting sense of satisfaction.

NOTE

1. The author would like to expression his thanks and appreciation for the supervision provided by Drs. Flora Hoodin, Ellen Koch, and Tamara Penix.

REFERENCES

Akhtar, S., & Thomson, J. A. (1982). Overview: Narcissistic personality disorder. *American Journal of Psychiatry, 139*, 12–20.

Eagle, M. N. (2000). A critical evaluation of current conceptions of transference and countertransference. *Psychoanalytic Psychology, 17*, 24–37.

Gabbard, G. O. (2000). *Psychodynamic psychiatry in clinical practice* (3rd ed.). Washington, DC: American Psychiatric Association.

Jacobs, T. (1991). *The use of the self*. Madison, CT: International Universities Press.

Jacobs, T. J. (1993). The inner experiences of an analyst: their contribution to the analytic process. *International Journal of Psycho-Analysis, 74*, 7–14.

Kernberg, O. F. (1967). Borderline personality organization. *Journal of American Psychoanalytic Association, 15*, 641–85.

Kohut, H. (1984). *How does analysis cure?* Chicago, IL: University of Chicago Press.

Kohut, H. (1968). The psychoanalytic treatment of narcissistic personality disorders. *Psychoanalytic Study of Children, 23*, 86–113.

Kohut, H. (1977). *The restoration of the self*. New York: International Universities.

Kohut, H. (1987). Value judgments surrounding narcissism. In M. Elson (Ed.), *The Kohut seminars on self psychology and psychotherapy with adolescents and young adults*. New York: Norton.

McWilliams, N. (1994). *Psychoanalytic diagnosis*. New York: Guilford.

Racker, H. (1968). *Transference and counter-transference*. NY: International University Press.

Wink, P. (1996). Narcissism. In C. G. Costello (Ed.), *Personality characteristics of the personality disordered*. New York: Guilford.

Wink, P. (1991). Two faces of narcissism. *Personality and Individual Differences, 33*, 379–91.

6

The Case of Mr. Edwards

Scott R. Brown[1]

CASE DESCRIPTION

Mr. Edwards was a thirty-eight-year-old Caucasian male who presented to a training clinic seeking help for two primary problems. First, Mr. Edwards was facing increasing distress due to his poor financial management, including increasing debt to both creditors and short-term loan agencies, such as advanced check-cashing locations. Second, he complained of increasing sexual frustration, due to his wife's inability to have sexual intercourse, because of surgery-related physiological changes. His wife was fifty-eight years old at the time of his intake.

Mr. Edwards's presentation was friendly, although his sense of social interaction seemed stilted. He would often make flippant or crude remarks about issues being discussed, and he often detailed graphic interest in pornographic materials. Despite these challenges during the rapport-building process, a strong alliance was constructed. Therapy focused initially on exploring the immediate presenting problems and determining the best course of treatment. It quickly became obvious that the presenting problems were intimately linked, both drawing from the patient's personal concept of what it meant to be a male. For Mr. Edwards, being a man meant being rich, successful, and sexually powerful.

Mr. Edwards worked in a white-collar office position, spending the majority of his time performing menial accounting procedures that he felt somewhat skilled at, but not overly enthused in pursuing. He believed that he was destined for greater success, meaning, as previously noted, that he would be rich, independently powerful, and realizing erotic fantasies. Much of our therapy work focused on discussing his job, the relationships at his workplace, his fantasies about business and success, and his plans for future employment (or the lack thereof). It gradually became clear that Mr. Edwards desired economic potency without any expended effort. He was continually drawn to "get-rich-quick" schemes, often based on absurd structures, tenets, and promises. However, the continued loss of money and failure at these prospects did not dissuade him from future attempts; in fact, it appeared that each loss of money and time bolstered his belief that he was "learning" and moving toward what would ultimately be millions of easily acquired dollars.

The most striking interpersonal feature that Mr. Edwards possessed was a seeming lack of understanding, or perhaps acceptance, of the norms that govern normal social interaction. Admittedly, while therapy is ideally supposed to elicit unfiltered emotions and interaction, it is still unusual for a patient to present the level of unabashed forwardness and explicitness that was evidenced during my first few sessions with Mr. Edwards. Not only would he openly express graphic sexual thoughts and behaviors, but also he would share his intimate troubles, including financial insecurity, with great candor. Further, throughout therapy, Mr. Edwards developed the habit of recounting stories or experiences many times, often seemingly verbatim from a script, without reference that these had been previously discussed. At first, it appeared that he was communicating in a stilted manner and relying on scripted responses to fill our time together; however, it gradually became evident that these were indeed genuine experiences for Mr. Edwards and, regardless of how well they reflected absolute reality, these accounts served as valid representations of Mr. Edwards's internal experiences throughout life, no matter how many times they were repeated or revisited. The repetition of such situations actually became very valuable from a clinical perspective, as it allowed for repeated and focused processing of details from Mr. Edwards's experiences. From a transference perspective, repeated visitations of key life experiences and situations allowed us to explore how Mr. Edwards related to individuals in his life and how these dynamics were being recreated in current problems or even in the therapy room.

For instance, Mr. Edwards would often discuss how his father had treated him while growing up and during his early adulthood; these descriptions were marked by feelings of frustration, shame, and low self-esteem—in essence, Mr. Edwards felt he "couldn't measure up." Further, it seemed that there were times during our sessions that he would try to meet what he perceived to be my expectations. By focusing on this dynamic, I was able to process Mr. Edwards's underlying feelings of shame and depleted narcissism, as well as the transference within the session—chiefly, that Mr. Edwards felt he needed to prove to me his worth and "measure up" to my standards, as he did with his father. Yet, Mr. Edwards's unwillingness to admit this process dynamic reflected his continued resistance to exploring his feelings surrounding his father and his own questions about self-worth and achievement.

It was the accumulation of the above traits and behaviors that gradually began to lead me and my supervisors to question the role of more dynamically-based character deficits in Mr. Edwards's presentation. His family history, his interpersonal relationships, his fantastical thinking about money and sex, and his preoccupation with material and libidinous power led us to consider whether Mr. Edwards was, at least in part, driven by narcissistic tendencies.[2]

Utilizing the hypothesis that Mr. Edwards possessed a narcissistic personality structure from a dynamic perspective allowed for treatment planning that included dynamic exploration of early experiences and attachment situations, as well as the role of process-related variables in therapy and in his interpersonal experiences. While this meant that we did not always focus on simple reductions in problem behaviors (e.g., investing in poor situations/schemes, social appropriateness), this tactic did allow for examination of the underlying motives responsible for continued engagement in these behaviors. Further, when warranted, more structured approaches were taken that allowed for direct comment on poor decision-making and possible problems that would severely affect the patient.

Mr. Edwards's treatment lasted for nearly three years. He was one of my first patients, and it is notable that I developed alongside him, growing more confident and comfortable in my new role. Indeed, although we often fail to admit such facts, our first patients, in some ways, do as much for us as we do for them. It was a positive experience for our treatment to last long enough for me to see incremental development and progress in Mr. Edwards; he endured changes that would challenge any of us, including the loss of his job, economic difficulties, and perhaps most difficult, the loss of his wife.

It should be noted that the current picture presented of Mr. Edwards is but a simple glimpse of the patient as a whole. Indeed, throughout psychological history, much of psychodynamic casework—and psychology casework, in general—is presented in such a manner, eliminating certain details and complexities in favor of anonymity and a constrained clinical focus. Therefore, I wish to acknowledge that the focus of this chapter is on narcissistic and other dynamic traits that the patient possessed; focusing on these areas limits the picture painted of the individual, who was markedly nuanced and complex, possessing at times striking compassion, insight, and emotionality. It would be remiss of us, as psychologists, to label our patients as simple objects or as possessors of traits, without always considering the depth and richness of their complete lives, although many of these seemingly irrelevant details are ignored both in textbooks and in therapy rooms. With that caveat, I proceed to detail some of the theoretical underpinnings important in examining Mr. Edwards's case.

THEORETICAL FOUNDATIONS

Before examining Mr. Edwards's historical background and development, it is important to discuss the basis for conceptualizing a core part of his treatment in terms of narcissistic characteristics. McWilliams (1994) describes narcissism very succinctly as "people whose personalities are organized around maintaining their self-esteem by getting affirmation from outside themselves" (p. 168). However, she is quick to note that this definition has been hotly debated since Freud first introduced the concept. Specifically, with the development of object relations theory in the middle part of the twentieth century, dynamic theory began to conceptualize narcissism as a form of compensation stemming from developmental deficits or conflicts with primary objects, such as the father or mother. By using a definition that addressed what was *lacking* in these individuals' lives, instead of seeing their behavior from a drive-based perspective, new methods of therapeutic intervention, such as mirroring (Winnicott, 1967; Schultz & Glickauf-Hughes, 1995; Kohut, 1968), could be utilized to actually treat narcissistic conflicts.

McWilliams (1994) also notes that the development of narcissistic personality often stems from a similar interaction with the parent or caregiver, wherein the child is utilized as a narcissistic extension, meaning that the child becomes the means of providing esteem and worth to the parent (see also, Miller, 1981). When this occurs, McWilliams (1994) argues that children become confused about who they are, given that their actions, performance, and identity stem solely from their relationship with a more powerful figure. In such situations, they necessarily need to seek out later their own affirmation from others and seek guidance from individuals who could protect and define them. With Mr. Edwards, this was evident (as will be briefly explored in the section on Mr. Edwards's history and background). Suffice it to say that his relationship with his parents, and especially his mother, always held an important place in his self-identity. When this relationship was disrupted by the introduction of other siblings who competed for his parents' attention, by private time between his parents, or by his personal development and maturation, he became distressed and lost. Indeed, one can see how his wife became a replacement for these early family members, serving as a compass and source of affirmation—in essence, reinstating his role as a narcissistic extension and fueling his own narcissistic energies.

It is important to note that there are two clearly delineated narcissistic personality types in dynamic theory (Gabbard, 2000). Wink (1991), Hotchkiss (2005), and McWilliams (1994) describe these as a devalued or depleted narcissism and a grandiose narcissism. Hotchkiss (2005) further explicates the distinction by using Kernberg's and Kohut's theories to illustrate the differences: specifically, she notes that "Kernberg's narcissist is someone in need of a moral tuneup, [while] Kohut's is a more pitiful character, a needy, depressed person with low self-esteem, a deep sense of uncared-for worthlessness and rejection, and a hunger for response and reassurance" (p. 131). Indeed, there is a schism of sorts within the dynamic community based upon the theories of Kernberg and Kohut. Kohut (1971, 1977) argued that narcissism represents a deflated ego and the inability of an individual to effectively relate to others without objectification and projection. For him, the goal was empathic understanding and mirroring of the patient's defenses and experiences, with the therapist becoming a curative influence by representing a completely novel relationship, wherein there was not judgment, expectation, or shame (Schultz & Glickauf-Hughes, 1995; Gabbard, 2000; McWilliams, 1994; Hotchkiss, 2005). Kernberg (1975, 1976, 1984) was more classically analytic in his style, arguing that narcissists must be confronted and challenged to reshape their interpersonal functioning and develop an understanding of relational dynamics (see also Gabbard, 2000).

To summarize the theory on narcissism that informs our exploration of Mr. Edwards's case, it is helpful to delineate the qualities that McWilliams (1994), Hotchkiss (2005), and Gabbard (2000) list as indicative of underlying narcissistic conflicts. First, there is a tendency to "split" within relationships, wherein another person or situation is idealized and subsequently devalued. Second, there is a propensity for grandiosity, although we have noted that the opposite experience of psychological identity depletion also is presented either covertly or manifestly. Third, there is a dramatic tendency toward feelings of shame and envy; it is important to note that these are emotions that require other people (i.e., self-objects) in order to exist. Shame is concerned with how we are seen by others, while envy is our reaction to that which others possess. Fourth, all three authors note that narcissism necessarily damages the patient's ability to actually love another and find meaning in such relationships. McWilliams (1994) states, "The most grievous cost of a narcissistic orientation is a stunted capacity to love" (p. 175).

Hotchkiss (2005) argues that narcissism is marked by immature and primitive defense mechanisms, such as denial, avoidance, and projection. These defenses, along with the inability to empathize with others, creates deficits in superego functioning, wherein narcissistic patients are unable to serve as their own moral compass and make judgments about the consequences of their actions. Finally, McWilliams (1994) makes particular comments about the presentation of narcissism in therapy, noting that patients with narcissistic conflicts are readily identifiable by our countertransference in session. Narcissists, she comments, have an ego-syntonic desire to use therapy as a means of perfecting themselves, instead of seeing it as a process of reflection, change, and development of coping techniques for continued struggles. This perspective, combined with the above-mentioned traits, creates strong and persistent countertransference, which will be explored in a later section.

Given the psychoanalytic or psychodynamic conceptualization of narcissistic personality, as explored above, I will examine the formative stage of the clinical relationship between Mr. Edwards and me. Mr. Edwards did not present as a DSM-IV-TR (APA, 2000) version of a narcissist—the type of person who believes whole-heartedly in his own superiority, espousing disdain and boredom with others, their interests, or the world at large, utilizing scathing comments and actions to defend against possible suggestions of inferiority. Instead, Mr. Edwards displayed a more subtle narcissism—a form of depleted narcissism, as mentioned previously.

During the formative stage of our relationship, I did not immediately believe that Mr. Edwards possessed the personality traits associated with narcissistic conflicts. Instead, his behaviors were suggestive of more basic psychological problems, perhaps even developmental delays or associated disorders. For instance, he would describe stories in an almost ritualized manner, each detail the same as a previous telling, and the perspective always decidedly first person. He displayed a marked deficit in his ability to relate to others, understand social norms, or utilize empathy to take another's perspective. Further, Mr. Edwards was unabashedly open about the inner workings of his mind and his drives: he would directly state his goals were to obtain money, sex, and charisma. I often would feel conflicted by Mr. Edwards's presentation during sessions: his candor, and the engagement in providing detailed background information, was endearing and helpful to a new therapist. However, this presentation was also socially unconventional, leading me to consider how he would appear in daily interpersonal interactions. In essence, while I found myself, as a therapist, intrigued and excited by Mr. Edwards's presentation, I was also able to understand how others would perceive him as immature and excessively blunt and how such individuals might take advantage of or mock him.

It was these feelings of compassion and concern I had for Mr. Edwards, in concert with some of his odd behaviors, which initially led my supervisor and me to consider developmental disabilities. However, his behaviors, upon further interaction and assessment, including the Minnesota Multiphasic Personality Inventory, 2nd Edition (MMPI-2), were found to be rooted more in personality traits that affected his ability to relate to others, understand societal norms, and ascertain his effect on others. In essence, it began to become obvious that he was, diagnostically, developmentally intact, insofar as he was not cognitively impaired; yet, it was clear that his development had led to the presentation of key character attributes that had contributed to his current problems and ongoing dynamic conflicts.

Indeed, each of the behaviors noted above as possibly indicative of developmental disability was explainable by various theorists' understanding of narcissistic conflict. The preoccupation with basic drives was clearly linked to inflated beliefs about self-worth and entitlement, while his self-centered storytelling provided evidence of his inability to relate to others, read social cues, and attend to norms. Further gathering of background information strengthened the argument for Mr. Edwards's narcissistic tendencies, as noted in the following section.

BACKGROUND INFORMATION

Mr. Edwards was raised in a relatively traditional family structure. His father worked as a salesman, who also was closely connected to the church, volunteering to help out at weekly services. Mr. Edwards was strongly influenced by Protestant religion during his development. In part this explains some of the thinking patterns in which he engaged, such as dichotomizing "good" and "evil" and believing that continual faith in a project, even if it is materially focused, will produce "magical," divinely-inspired results; in a way, Mr. Edwards felt "worthy" of success and believed that a Higher Power should ennoble him with wealth and power.

Mr. Edwards's mother was very close to him during development, although the birth of other children forced her to split her attention, causing some conflict within Mr. Edwards. He never spoke explicitly of the relationship between him and his parents before the birth of his other siblings, although he clearly presented a sense of having a close, special connection, especially with his mother. This special connection was also apparent later in Mr. Edwards's life, and during our work together, when Mr. Edwards reported calling his mother frequently, praying with her every morning and evening, and visiting her several times a week. He admitted that he was somewhat jealous of the attention granted to his siblings, especially attention his father gave his youngest brother. At one point in his adolescence, Mr. Edwards indicated that he "tested" his parents' capacity to help and care for him with a bullying situation at school (i.e., a peer was picking on him); he indicated they failed to help him by making him stand on his own in the situation. Specifically, he said that they refused to act on his behalf and speak with the bully, the bully's parents, or school officials; he said that they told him to stand up for himself and take care of the situation. Mr. Edwards reports that this was a strong blow to the connection he felt with his parents, especially his mother. He indicated that he saw this as his mother allying with his father, instead of advocating for his best interests and needs.

A key reason for Mr. Edwards's perceived rejection at the hands of his parents was the arrival of several other children in the family, of whom

Mr. Edwards was the oldest. Mr. Edwards had two other siblings, both male. One brother (the older of the two) was a successful businessman, who seemed to possess high levels of intellect and compassion. Mr. Edwards seemed to admire this brother and possess underlying wishes to emulate him; however, mixed with these positive feelings were twinges of jealousy and coveting. In a way, this brother seemed to have assimilated the mantle of their father. Mr. Edwards would often discuss this brother when trying to determine whether an employment decision for himself was useful or wise.

Mr. Edwards did not provide significant detail into his relationship with his youngest brother, perhaps because he was the only sibling who was deceased. He had died in his twenties in a car accident. The most concrete comment Mr. Edwards provided regarding his brother was that "he got plenty of sex." This comment was a striking example of the often blunt and rather immature thought processes that Mr. Edwards engaged in; further, the comment represents Mr. Edwards's fantasies regarding power and sex, in that pleasure and satisfaction are determine by one's prowess and engagement in sexual interactions.

In addition to his relationships with his siblings, Mr. Edwards often described his cousin, who was a completely different type of individual than his brothers; this relative was a continual failure in Mr. Edwards's eyes, not just in business and financial matters—but since he was gay—in life as a whole. Mr. Edwards, in his more insightful and genuine moments, would sometimes admit to being afraid that he identified with this cousin, if only in matters of his lack of financial success. Interestingly, Mr. Edwards spent a significant amount of time in his life fighting claims that he was gay. He would continually tell stories in session about his father confronting him after he was married, claiming that he was gay. Mr. Edwards quickly assured me, and himself, that he was heterosexual, as evidenced by his love of sex and his fantasies about women. He claimed that his mother originally sided with his father but, after his father's death, that she told him she knew he was not gay. Mr. Edwards's anxiety surrounding sexuality was considered at various points in treatment; however, he minimized it and would quickly utilize psychological defenses to avoid discussion of the topic, such as denial and, at a more sophisticated level, reaction formation, wherein he became hypermasculine and oversexualized, describing his heterosexual fantasies and experiences in graphic, often crude, detail. Therefore, it remained a relatively unexamined aspect of his psyche.

One of the most salient and powerful figures in Mr. Edwards's life was his wife. Margaret was significantly senior in years to Mr. Edwards and nearly the same age as his mother. In many ways, she was a mother figure for Mr. Edwards. He continually denied that she guided him or "mothered" him, but their interactions clearly marked a relationship shaped not simply by traditional romantic mores, but by childlike attention- and guidance-seeking. Mr. Edwards and Margaret seemed to both offer each other something the other needed—one needed guidance, warmth, and a strong conscience, while the other sought appreciation, youth, and hope. In this light, their relationship was strikingly endearing and powerful. However, Margaret also became his most powerful self-object, fulfilling his needs to bolster his ego, fuel his grandiose fantasies, and make some progress on proving his masculinity and power to his father, who was critical and judgmental of his son's sexual identity and life. In addition, it seemed that Margaret utilized Mr. Edwards as a form of narcissistic extension, in that she thrived on his achievements and fantasies. Indeed, she had found a much younger man with some promise in his work and life; for her, his world became hers and gave her youth, vitality, and, as evidenced by Mr. Edwards's comments, sexuality. This complex bond, wherein his narcissism and her extension of him as an aspect of her identity became entwined, reenacted for Mr. Edwards the childhood attention he had received and lost.

As evidenced by Mr. Edwards's preference for interactions with older, maternal figures, it became clear that he was uncomfortable in social or familial situations with adult male peers. Indeed, same-sex social situations in general always had been difficult for Mr. Edwards. He described only one childhood friend, with whom he lost contact after high school. His father reportedly belittled their relationship, making comments and jokes that Mr. Edwards took to mean that he and his friend were gay. During high school, Mr. Edwards reported that he had no romantic involvement. In fact, the only concrete sexual experience Mr. Edwards described during high school was a fantasy involving a female classmate in a gym class propositioning him by simply making eye contact while he ran around the track. The lack of actual evidence that she was interested in him, even when he admitted that he did not know her, was no deterrent to his continued belief that she wanted him to have sex with her. In fact, these types of sexual fantasies, marked by a lack of basis in reality and possessing almost pornographic themes, were presented consistently, throughout therapy. The high school incident along with several situations involving a select group of others were the most often-referenced fantasies.

Mr. Edwards was not socially active during college. He reported that he had his first girlfriend in college and that he "could've had sex with her," but he decided not to. His description of this experience wavered at times, and it was always unclear whether his lack of sexual involvement with the girlfriend reflected a lack of desire on her part or his. After their break-up near the end of college, Mr. Edwards began a period of relatively unfocused living. He lived with his parents for a time, shifting from job to job, although he had been trained in accounting. He described this period largely by recounting experiences in adult clubs and his viewing of erotic movies.

At this time, Mr. Edwards still had not had sexual intercourse, so these outlets were a surrogate for him, reflecting the immense internal conflict surrounding his libido and, indeed, his struggling identity. His developing desire for power and money led him to investigate for the first time self-empowerment seminars and programs. It was through these experiences that he eventually discovered Margaret, who would become his wife. In sessions he carefully described how he had decided that he wanted to marry an older, mature, sexually experienced woman. And, when making most references to his wife in therapy sessions, he would affirm that they had had a wonderful sexual life and that his wife possessed a nearly insatiable sexual appetite. Mr. Edwards failed to develop insight into the defenses against his sense of insecurity as evidenced by these statements. These included rationalization and denial of his insecurities with younger women and his desire for an older woman, who in many ways represented a mother figure to which he had never felt close enough—even though he and his mother had shared periods of close contact and mutual support— as well as a person who could reinstate the narcissistic extension he desired.

In many ways, the most potent and formative figure for Mr. Edwards remained his father. Although he seemed to have sought out a mother-figure, and remained close to his mother throughout his life, it became evident that his father had taken on an almost deity-like role in Mr. Edwards's psyche. He often was outwardly disdainful of his father's perceived manipulation and deceit, but Mr. Edwards would also soften these words with underlying awe and jealousy. He even agreed that he "couldn't measure up" to his father's standards. Mr. Edwards would often describe his father as a salesman—a trait he seemed to have used effectively in his work—who could change his mood and presentation at will, selling to attentive others his story and position. Mr. Edwards seemed to feel that his father was often disingenuous, including a time when his father came to him after a prolonged separation between them (spurred on by his father's accusations that he was gay) and asked him to come back to the family. Mr. Edwards described this experience as artificial and troubling, but he was not able to resist his father's appeals. Eventually, he reconnected with him. In many ways, Mr. Edwards's father represented the epitome of his concept of a successful man: a persuasive smooth-talker who possessed charisma and charm, a financially stable (although not overly successful) individual who also had a sex life that Mr. Edwards overtly fantasized was potent and exciting. It became increasingly clear in treatment that Mr. Edwards's quest for masculine power was an effort to secure a position equal or greater to that of his father, and perhaps prove once and for all to his father that he was a strong, competent, secure heterosexual male. Therefore, one can see Mr. Edwards's psychological conflict, wherein his narcissism and self-involvement were fueled by incessant insecurities.

TREATMENT HISTORY

Mr. Edwards's treatment began somewhat awkwardly, since it was unclear how best to help him address his presenting problems. While frank and blunt about his perceived problems with sexuality, Mr. Edwards quickly minimized the importance of these issues after intake, instead spending the majority of the first few assessment and intake sessions discussing his workplace, job security, and financial difficulties. In fact, both my supervisor and I noted that the issues he believed were most important seemed better served by a financial planner. Mr. Edwards met this idea, however, with reservation and defensiveness. It appeared that Mr. Edwards possessed some sense of the failures he was experiencing with finances, but that he could not change these behaviors simply by being told what to do; instead, at some level he was seeking to address underlying fears, insecurities, and intrapersonal conflicts that drove him to continue engaging in these activities and making poor decisions that impacted his well-being.

It is important to note that the clinic at which I saw Mr. Edwards utilized various theoretical modalities, including psychodynamic, cognitive behavioral therapy (CBT), solution-focused, and interpersonal techniques. Given that Mr. Edwards appeared to be spinning out of control at intake, in terms of his financial well-being, the initial treatment plan was to focus on how Mr. Edwards planned to address his financial issues. Our theoretical assumption was that Mr. Edwards would be amenable to a solution-focused approach, wherein his past experiences and successes could shape the solution to the current problem. However, a key problem became evident when exploring this idea: Mr. Edwards had never truly found solutions to problems. Instead, he seemed to compound them with short-term or ineffective solutions. When in serious financial trouble, Mr. Edwards had used bankruptcy, questionable tax maneuvers, and even resorted to manipulating family and social contacts to raise money under false pretenses. While these had, in some ways, "fixed" the immediate problem, they clearly did not solve the longer range problems, and they did not promote Mr. Edwards's psychological health and sense of self-efficacy.

Therefore, I began to explore what was motivating him to continue investment in risky areas and businesses. The first three to six months of treatment were aimed at better understanding Mr. Edwards's perspective on money and wealth, along with continual monitoring of his financial behaviors. Further, I encouraged him to begin questioning his investment decisions and move toward reducing his losses. I suggested to him that doing so, while perhaps not as gratifying as "instant wealth," would help him develop a sense of achievement and success. In addition, he would be able to focus more on work tasks—an area he admitted to neglecting—and improve his performance there, helping others notice him and appreciate his contribution. While a seemingly simple form of treatment, these interactions proved very useful. Toward the end of the six-month period, Mr. Edwards had successfully paid off several debts and ceased involvement in many risky plans. Indeed, he had a period of investment "sobriety," wherein he avoided spending any money in questionable schemes and, when he was engaging in negative investment behaviors, these expenditures were limited to one or two new "businesses" at a time. This was marked progress for Mr. Edwards.

Even further progress was achieved by asking Mr. Edwards to conceptualize his investment behaviors as a form of gambling addiction. I sought out some form of conceptualization tool because I increasingly felt as though Mr. Edwards required a more concrete definition or understanding of his problems. In hindsight, it is notable that Mr. Edwards seemed to be creating a transferential relationship markedly similar to dynamics he engaged in with his parents, specifically his father, wherein he sought to have others tell him what was the right or wrong choice and to guide him through difficult decisions or situations (e.g., the bullying situation described previously, where Mr. Edwards "tested" his parents' willingness to help and comfort him). Therefore, while reviewing the case at the six-month mark, I noted that the DSM-IV-TR (APA, 2000) definition of pathological gambling was remarkably similar to the behaviors Mr. Edwards presented. I reworded the definition to include "investment schemes" for words referring to gambling and read the DSM-IV-TR description to him. Mr. Edwards was taken aback and agreed that this indeed did fit his view of such behaviors and his continued engagement in risky investments. Since my supervisor at the time had significant experience with gambling-related treatments, we agreed to introduce a modified, cognitive behavioral protocol for gambling treatment and asked Mr. Edwards, on a weekly basis, to explore a new topic related to gambling and completing worksheets in-session. However, Mr. Edwards's interactions in therapy and his overall demeanor shifted noticeably—it appeared he was holding back. This much more structured, cognitive-behavioral technique chilled our alliance. As I look back on the treatment, the reasons for such a reaction are clear, given the personality dynamics inherent in Mr. Edwards's presentation. By focusing treatment on structured tasks and assignments, I eliminated the reinforcing function I had been serving as Mr. Edwards's self-object. In response, he pulled away, unsure of how to relate to me when I was not serving such a function.

In light of the father-like transference noted above, it is also likely that Mr. Edwards experienced this interaction as excessively didactic, perhaps even as scolding. Prior to focusing on the problem and attempting to "teach" Mr. Edwards the best means of dealing with his problems, Mr. Edwards was experiencing me as an idealized version of a father-figure, one who accepted him, praised even incremental progress, and allowed him to explore his problems in a safe, corrective relationship. Therefore, the gambling protocol made little contribution to treatment, and it was terminated several weeks later. It appeared that Mr. Edwards developed surface insight into his problem (i.e., conceptualizing it as a form of gambling and addiction), but he remained unwilling to deepen this insight by engaging in targeted worksheets or modules. In fact, his behaviors in-session were more confrontational and defensive; he was clearly using defense mechanisms to protect against perceived attacks to his ego.

It became evident that while surface progress was made on addressing the presenting complaints, there existed significant underlying psychological conflict and distress. Further, it seemed that such distress was linked to personality characteristics and rigid ways of thinking. Exploring these qualities and beginning to address the underlying dynamics that might be shaping his current situation seemed a valuable therapeutic shift, especially given the relative stability of his financial situation at that point in treatment.

Psychotherapy became more dynamically-based, using current problems and difficulties as a means to explore long-standing behaviors, especially as these related to his view of "success" and "achievement." Mr. Edwards was amenable to this shift, which included increased depth of emotional processing in-session and the use of interpretation, developmental experiences, and interpersonal dynamics as a means to understanding long-standing behaviors.

During our increasingly dynamic therapy, Mr. Edwards presented the behaviors and dynamics that cemented my conceptualization of his narcissistic conflicts. The shift to dynamic treatment provided a sort of ambiguous stimulus or environment for Mr. Edwards. I believe that this was compounded by the more reserved approach I took in-session; I utilized a more analytic demeanor, wherein I did not immediately educate on or interpret the material that was brought up. Instead, I used these instances to process Mr. Edwards's emotions and developmental experiences, in addition to simple reflection of underlying themes. This ambiguity during session, combined with me not providing Mr. Edwards concrete guidance or judgment, aided in uncovering many of his defense mechanisms. When pressed to focus on certain issues, emotions, or experiences, and to connect these to previously discussed topics or developmental issues, Mr. Edwards became clearly reactive, stating that he was feeling "bullied" or pressured by the therapist and denying any connection. He was careful to note his appreciation for the therapist's expertise, hard work, and caring, but he avoided these topics, nonetheless.

As can be derived from this limited description of this treatment period, it was a time of conflict and struggle, during which Mr. Edwards's narcissism became most apparent. He continued to articulate libidinous desires linked to underlying feelings of grandiosity and entitlement; indeed, his goals

(wealth, power, sex—in essence, omnipotence) remained excessively infantile and unsophisticated. Mr. Edwards's openness and the more dynamic-
based processing of these issues drew these characteristics to the surface. At
one point, Mr. Edwards shared his belief that if he successfully sold prod-
ucts for one new investment, he would have a box of one-hundred dollar
bills delivered by hand to his house. The absurdity and impracticality of this
belief was ignored fully by Mr. Edwards. For him, the fantasy was so powerful it overpowered reason and, from a dynamic perspective, the simplistic
fantasy suited his undeveloped, immature psyche.

Mr. Edwards engaged in *splitting* during sessions. I was often the target of
both idealization as well as demonization. When I supported his growth,
his insight, and his progress, he would paint a picture of me as a friend,
confidant, and close ally. Further, during these times of idealization, I became to Mr. Edwards a wonderfully insightful and experienced clinician,
addressing his issues with skill and panache. However, one slight challenge,
question, or interpretation could change these attributions; within moments, I could become "a bully" who was attacking not just his behaviors,
but it would seem, his very being. While Mr. Edwards would lash out to defend in the moment, he had to repair his alliance for at least two reasons:
one, I represented an ideal self, who he seemed to believe was successful in
the areas he considered important (wealth, intelligence, sexuality, and
power), and a father-like figure who judged him but also cared for him;
eliminating that alliance would devastate his need for such a self-object.
Second, at times it seemed as though he viewed us as equals, his narcissism
buoying his self-esteem and confidence to a point that there was often the
feeling, if not subtle verbalizations, that Mr. Edwards viewed us as "friends."
I believe that he thought repairing the alliance through idealization would
eliminate future threats from me challenging him in session and lead me to
serve a self-object purpose, reflecting his idealization of me onto him.

Mr. Edwards also would utilize splitting with others in his life. Mr. Edwards would clearly articulate how close he had become to certain people
at work and how warmly he felt toward them, as long as they helped him
with projects and tasks. When they affronted him, or if he even perceived
such actions, he quickly expressed disdain for them and their competence.
His manipulations of them are interesting to note. Mr. Edwards would commonly state that he did little things, like buy them a newspaper or compliment them, in order to garner their favor and help. It was clear, from a
moral perspective, that Mr. Edwards had not internalized such deeds as caring and compassionate; instead, his motives were purely self-serving,
thereby strengthening my narcissistic conceptualization of his case.

Finally, Mr. Edwards began to increasingly utilize defensive mechanisms
during treatment. Most of these were immature defenses, such as simple denial or avoidance, projection, and, at the upper-echelon of Mr. Edwards's

defensive hierarchy, rationalization. As Hotchkiss (2005) noted, narcissistic personality types will tend to use these forms of defensiveness, partly because of their lack of ability to relate to others and also as a result of their fixation, at some level, to an earlier, infantile, developmental stage. Much as a child or infant will whine, cry, hit, or scream to avoid unpleasant stimuli, Mr. Edwards used basic defenses to avoid uncomfortable topics and emotions. Helping him realize these defenses, and perhaps other means of dealing with negative stimuli, was a core part of therapy.

It should be noted that the conflict and defensiveness observed in session were not necessarily a negative therapeutic factor. These conflicts and struggles marked an important beginning for Mr. Edwards, wherein he began to explore his own identity and the relationships he had developed throughout his life. By focusing on these issues, and the dynamic of the therapist-patient dyad itself, he was able to begin developing increased insight into the underlying problems that led to his initial presentation. Therapy during this period was not always easy or explicitly enjoyable; however, it was a valuable shift that I believe helped Mr. Edwards make significant progress. Further, while Mr. Edwards was reticent to explore many of these areas, he was fully engaged in treatment; he rarely missed a session and commented that he looked forward to our meetings. For Mr. Edwards, the therapy room and our relationship remained a safe place to explore his problems, although these issues now involved more focused processing of difficult emotions and experiences.

However, there were times of tension within the session. In one session, Mr. Edwards began discussing how he wanted to be wealthy and powerful— a topic that was broached most sessions. I noticed a feeling of frustration and boredom, reflecting the feeling of "spinning our wheels" that is common with narcissistic patients, as noted by McWilliams (1994). I chose to attempt an interpretation. I asked him if his continued obsession with money, power, and sex reflected something we had previously discussed, mainly that he never felt he could "measure up" to his father's expectations. Mr. Edwards's reaction was automatic. He vaulted forward in his seat slightly and pointed a finger at me, exclaiming, "You're being a bully!" We explored this reaction, and he seemed to remain incensed for a period of several minutes. He then quickly returned to idealizing me, seemingly in an attempt to remove the focus on him. He did report later in session, near the conclusion of our meeting, that the office space reminded him of a German prison interrogation room. The significance of such a comment is clear, although he denied the suggestion that he was feeling like a prisoner being pushed for information. In hindsight, it is clear that this interpretation, while likely accurate and thereby leading to Mr. Edwards's powerful reaction, was "too much, too fast."

During our last year together, Mr. Edwards experienced an enormously life-changing event, which would become a core focus of therapy: his wife died. This event was relatively unexpected. She died from acute respiratory failure resulting from complications with the flu. Within one week of being admitted to the hospital, she died. As can be expected from such an event, processing her death was difficult and meaningful for Mr. Edwards, especially given his relative social isolation and the nature of their relationship. Mr. Edwards's wife was a friend and, in many ways, a mother-figure. She was near his mother's age, so her passing served as a reminder of mortality in general, specifically causing him to worry about how long he would have his mother nearby. Perhaps more importantly, from a dynamic perspective, was that Mr. Edwards's wife served as an important self-object that helped fulfill unmet narcissistic needs from his childhood. With his wife, he was able to use her to bolster his own esteem, while having her guide him and use his own internalized grandiosity to fuel her personal functioning and identity. They were entwined in a particularly complex manner, and her passing meant that Mr. Edwards was suddenly without his most valuable means of self-reflection and empowerment.

Mr. Edwards's narcissism was clearly active during these months as well. While he presented with visible grief and what I believe to be genuine sadness, the roots of these emotions were unclear. He quickly would shift subjects and often even appeared happy in session, discussing his plans for the future and his desire to find another woman. In addition, the sudden boon of his wife's small life insurance policy began to rekindle his interest in "get-rich-quick" schemes. This reaction is not surprising when considering them as defensive reactions against the devastation Mr. Edwards felt internally. However, his callousness and lack of a genuine grieving period were evident not only in the therapy room, but also in the broader world and with other individuals who were less able to understand the intricacies of his behavior and the grief underlying his actions.

I remember one specific discussion, approximately two to three weeks after his wife's passing, when Mr. Edwards began the session by detailing his wife's funeral and his interactions with family. At first, he appeared quiet, withdrawn, and contemplative. He was alone and he felt helpless at times. I was struck by his insight and his openness as he explained how he was unable to do things around the house as well without her. It was the simple things that he seemed to miss, the kind of things one may take for granted in a long-term partnership. I encouraged him to explore these emotions more, as a core part of our therapy at this point was for him to begin moving beyond intellectualization and into feelings. He began his description of the funeral in this mindset, articulating his emotions and the compassion he received from others. Then, he noted, rather flippantly, that he had shared with several other funeral attendees, including his brother, that he now planned to find another woman. In our session, he explained that he was excited to have sex again. It is likely that these over-sexualized thoughts and desires provided a defense against the intense emotions he was experiencing. The profound loss of his wife—a very powerful and tangible love-object—likely led Mr. Edwards to feel pain and confusion he had not previously experienced.

He clearly did not understand the social taboos and norms regarding mourning and loss. In one sense, her passing and the sudden increase in his libido-driven behavior confirmed an earlier hypothesis that she acted as part of his internalized conscience, much as I believe I had become. Without this guidance and the reminder of his superego, Mr. Edwards was in a sense unbridled and allowed to begin earnestly pursuing his drives. Further, it is likely that these drives defended against the pain of her loss. Therapy at this time focused on exploring these drives, processing their roots and development, and attempting to find means of appropriately expressing them. Further, our own relationship continued to serve as a valuable source of information about Mr. Edwards's dynamic interactions and underlying process variables that influenced his day-to-day life.

Toward the conclusion of our treatment, in the last four to six months, the focus of our work became Mr. Edwards's productivity and employment, due to the sudden loss of his accountant position at the firm for which he had worked nearly ten years. Mr. Edwards was warned of the job loss and able to prepare himself mentally for the shift; however, I believe he was unprepared for the emotions that came with his unemployment. After losing his wife, he had reinvested himself in work, perhaps unconsciously, and developed stronger bonds with workplace staff, since they were his only social outlets. The loss of these relationships and the sense of purpose he felt at work placed Mr. Edwards on the brink of serious depression. However, Mr. Edwards's defenses and emotional avoidance served as psychological safety nets. For Mr. Edwards, the job loss was rationalized as a temporary failure and, eventually, seen as an opening or opportunity for him to explore his full economic potential, although seriously limiting his social interaction.

Unfortunately, his "full economic potential" meant a radical increase in risky financial investments and schemes. Mr. Edwards's narcissism revolved around the definition of being male that I mentioned earlier: being rich, successful, and sexually powerful. With the loss of his job and his wife, two of these fantasies had suffered serious setbacks. He was left with a sole outlet for his narcissism and his libidinous energies: wealth. Therefore, our treatment moved toward exploring the roots of this desire for wealth and the emotions that surrounded this quest. Further, I moved toward increasingly structured sessions, focusing on concrete variables, wherein we examined his recent decisions, and I tried to influence him to care for himself by not risking too much money. While he was able to make gains in this area, I became a stabilizing object, empathically assuaging his fears while giving advice and guidance that I could only hope would be internalized.

As my training at the psychology clinic was ending, we concluded treatment together in a positive fashion. We spent a significant amount of time exploring our separation in session, although Mr. Edwards never admitted to any underlying feelings of loss, apart from statements about how helpful I had been and how he respected me. While Mr. Edwards agreed to see a therapist at an outside agency, it remained unclear whether he was invested fully in the exploration of his identity enough to commit to a long-term dynamic program of therapy beyond that which we had completed. Indeed, several months after our termination, through contact with his new therapist (Mr. Edwards had signed a release at termination), I learned that Mr. Edwards had dropped out of treatment after about two months of weekly sessions. The therapist explained that attempts to directly confront Mr. Edwards produced defensiveness and, eventually, seemed to lead to early termination. I also wondered what role the loss of our relationship played in his termination, especially in regards to my role as a transferential figure and self-object. The new therapist did not have any follow-up information on Mr. Edwards since he left their clinic.

It should be noted that Mr. Edwards never fully achieved the insight for which I hoped. This is not to say I was disappointed in his progress. Quite the contrary, I was often amazed and pleased by the gains he made in admitting his problems and the concrete strides he made in improving his life. Still, it was clear, especially near the end of our treatment together, that the insight concerning his behavior and the root of his inadequacies (perhaps their very presence) was poorly integrated into his self-concept: Mr. Edwards made tenuous progress that was noticeable chiefly when circumstances allowed him to solve tangible problems. For instance, during the portion of treatment that we focused on financial well being (roughly the first half of our three year relationship), Mr. Edwards became acquainted with a family friend who had reportedly endured similar hardship financially. This individual offered to help him pay off loans and move toward a more secure situation, although he would have to pay back this person. He realized the potential of this offer, took him up on his charity, and paid him back in approximately a year. Mr. Edwards made a positive decision and successfully avoided falling into the loan trap for the remainder of our work together. However, it was clear that he saw this as a means to avoid harm, not as a means to improve his financial and emotional well-being. In many ways, this was the conundrum of therapy with Mr. Edwards: his poorly integrated sense of self and the rawness of his narcissistic desires led to poorly controlled outlets for his behaviors. It appeared that only through external controls such as his mother, his wife, or myself (all, in essence, surrogate super-egos), could Mr. Edwards temper his drives and reduce his poor decision-making. While he made minor progress in internalizing these relationships, it remained a core component of treatment until we ended treatment together.

In sum, I look back on my therapeutic work with Mr. Edwards with feelings of satisfaction and disappointment. I believe that we worked together through difficult issues, made significant gains on practical problems, and began to delve deeper into his personality. However, I think that Mr. Edwards never successfully integrated fully our progress into his own identity and his relational dynamics. For instance, the most progress we made on parsing apart the roles of the super-ego, id, and ego and moving toward a more integrated sense of self was a caricatured version of psychological functioning wherein Mr. Edwards was caught between his internal "devil," telling him to take risks, and an externalized version of myself as superego, asking him what the risks entailed and whether he had examined the possible consequences of his actions. Further, after his wife's death, it seemed that he clearly lost some of his decision-making abilities and self-restraint. While his wife had contributed in some ways to previous risks and problems, it seemed that the dialogue the two shared served Mr. Edwards as a means of reflecting on the situation, determining the risks inherent in a situation, and moving toward at least a less damaging outcome than one made without external input.

COUNTERTRANSFERENCE

Schultz and Glickauf-Hughes (1995) noted that it is often through our countertransference reactions that we first identify personality dynamics and associated problems in our patients. This is especially true for cases of narcissistic pathology (Schultz & Glickauf-Hughes, 1995; McWilliams, 1994). With Mr. Edwards, my countertransference became an important tool that I used to assess our progress, our alliance, and my own reactions to the process of therapy. As noted by McWilliams (1994), the form of transference we see from narcissistic patients is much different from that seen in other contexts. Their limited empathy and their intense self-focus makes their own experience of transference and object relatedness complex and difficult. However, this reluctance to address process, and the process of therapy itself, elicits very strong and marked reactions in the therapist.

As noted previously, my experience with Mr. Edwards, as I believe is true of all our patients, was varied and marked by many different emotions and thoughts, including very positive feelings of pride in Mr. Edwards's progress, happiness, grief, and humor. That said, it is very true that my time with Mr. Edwards produced reactions unlike those felt with most of my other patients, especially in that these emotions did remain relatively static and unchanging, reflecting the rigidity of thought and relatedness present in narcissistic pathology.

I began consciously focusing on countertransference a few months into treatment, when we began to move into directly addressing his financial problems and, underneath this work, began moving toward exploration of long-term dynamics and patterns that resulted in his desire for material and libidinal outlets. There are at least two reasons why countertransference became the focus of my attention at this point in treatment. First, our initial work focused on surface exploration of Mr. Edwards's presenting complaints, much as is done with any patient. Second, and perhaps more important, was my lack of attention to process-related variables. During the beginning of our treatment, as noted previously, our work focused on more structured, supportive exploration of Mr. Edwards's financial problems and everyday struggles, including some cognitive behavioral techniques. Later on, however, it became obvious that in order to make more progress on these issues, as well as underlying dynamic problems—such as Mr. Edwards's depleted narcissism—we had to focus on the process variables in session. This exploration of process-related variables was also recommended by my supervisor. While earlier supervisors, including those who focused on more structured treatment modalities, were generally open to discussion of my reactions to the patient and process variables in the session, the switch to a strongly psychodynamic supervisor during this middle phase provided the impetus to focus even more intensely on these factors during treatment.

While I understood the concepts of transference, countertransference, and related variables, utilizing these tools and understanding the true import of attending to my own thoughts and feelings was relatively new to me and allowed me to develop my clinical skills in ways I had not realized they could develop. It seemed to me that, as new therapists early in our training, we struggle to remember the basics, such as intake procedures, charting duties, and treatment planning. As time and experience continue, we become more comfortable with complex clinical techniques and conceptualizations that are the product of sitting in the therapy room, building bonds, and dealing comfortably with crises and distress. In the case of Mr. Edwards, by the time we moved toward a dynamic focus in therapy, I felt more confident and comfortable as a therapist, especially in dealing with the more personal and often emotionally charged issues of process and the therapist-patient dyad. That said, I do believe that earlier and greater attention to dynamic variables, such as transference and countertransference, would have been helpful in my work with Mr. Edwards. Though I now realize that skill development and theoretical diversity in training and supervision affected when and how dynamic variables became more the focus of my work with Mr. Edwards, it seems to me that therapists should move toward inclusion of these variables as early as possible in treatment.

I noticed strong countertransference experiences during the middle phase of therapy. Mainly, I became very bored, often finding my mind wandering and counting the minutes until we were "finished." McWilliams (1994) reported that this is very common with such patients, noting that therapists will often feel drained, bored, and drowsy during sessions. She even explained how she had experienced this phenomenon, initially ascribing it to a large meal, a late appointment, or other mundane explanations. However, after having several patients in a row and finding that the drowsiness was only present with narcissistic patients, she began to understand the true countertransference behind such experiences. Schultz and Glickauf-Hughes (1995) describe this reaction as a direct result of the patient's own "mirror transference," wherein "the therapist is likely to have the experience of not being acknowledged by the client as a separate being" (p. 602). In essence, I began to become simply a self-object used by Mr. Edwards for gratification of his narcissistic personality structure.

In between sessions, I would begin to worry about the next session, in a sense dreading the hour with Mr. Edwards, as I perceived it. I could not definitively determine the roots of this reaction. And while Mr. Edwards and I always had some meaningful discourse and discussion in his sessions, it admittedly never involved deep exploration of his insight into his pathology, his current problems, or his relationships. I dealt with this reaction by consulting with my supervisor. As we explored this reaction, it became clear that while the sessions were generally "full" of content, they contained little else: specifically, I began to experience the tension between process and content, wherein we had plenty of material to explore—that is, details about weekly or daily happening with coworkers, relatives, or investment opportunities—but little focus on the dynamic processes inherent in these situations or, indeed, within the session itself. Further, Mr. Edwards continually defended against attempts on my part to refocus on the process. I spent several sessions delineating the therapeutic frame, as it related to process variables. I informed Mr. Edwards about the meaning of process and what was important to focus on when exploring these variables, including his emotional reaction to experiences with others, including myself. While he indicated understanding and assent to the technique, within a short period of time Mr. Edwards was retelling stories and situations we had previously explored, but without insight into these experiences or into the therapeutic process itself. I wanted more—chiefly, for Mr. Edwards to make some gains during the course of treatment that were noticeable and concrete, and to which he could ascribe some level of insight. His intense self-focus limited his ability to process such situations in a novel light, especially his ability to see something from another's perspective. Further, attempts to delve deeper into a topic or to address new topics through redirection resulted in retreat by Mr. Edwards, either through blatant denial or subtly more sophisticated defensive mechanisms. For instance, Mr. Edwards would often attempt to diffuse conflict during session and redirect a topic by glorifying my experience, insight, and aptitude as a clinician—another common form of countertransference seen with narcissistic patients (Schultz & Glickauf-Hughes, 1995). It seemed that he thought by projecting his own self-inflated image on me that he could feed my own narcissism; I believe that his specific goal in these instances was to idealize me, while minimize the focus on him during our explorations. I represented an ideal self, who he seemed to believe was successful in the areas he considered important (wealth, intelligence, sexuality, and power), and a father-like figure who judged him but also cared for him; eliminating that alliance would devastate his need for such a self-object. In effect, these entreaties only resulted in me becoming more bored and frustrated, feeling that the session had become a superficial exchange of compliments and devoid of true purpose.

As our dynamic therapy work progressed and my countertransference experiences became more apparent, I consulted with a local psychoanalyst who agreed to review the case, watch a session on tape, and discuss underlying themes and ideas in a group supervision setting. This supervision and consultation were both fascinating and useful; it confirmed my own conceptualization and added some thoughts on the process of our sessions. Specifically, this consultant noted that Mr. Edwards was avoidant of his own defensive processes and emotions, in general. However, more importantly, the analyst commented on my own countertransference and provided some guidance on addressing these feelings throughout our continued treatment.

A key part of this countertransference—the idea of being used as a self-object—elicited feelings of frustration and, in a sense, violation. I explored this in-depth during supervision, focusing on my feelings that I was not really needed in session and that Mr. Edwards was "running the show," utilizing me solely as a sounding board and as a form of paid "friend." My supervisor noted that this was common with narcissistic patients, in that their lack of empathic connection with others limited the tangibility of the alliance during sessions. Further, he noted that mirroring, to a limited degree, was what Kohut (1968, 1971, 1977) described in his treatment of narcissistic pathology. By engaging the individual in a novel relationship, reflecting and mirroring their emotions, providing the empathy and insight they lacked, and by subtly avoiding simplification into a self-object or extension of the patient, the therapist can create a corrective experience, leading to gradual gains in insight and empathy by the patient. My supervisor noted that Kernberg (1975, 1976, 1984) advocated more direct challenges and interpretation, but we both felt this seemed ill-suited for Mr. Edwards, as evidenced by my exploration of a challenge during session which I described earlier in the chapter. Mr. Edwards avoided challenges at all costs, reflecting his depleted form of narcissism, as opposed to the more emotionally charged grandiose-type. Without an identifiable emotional reaction that provides important clues to therapeutic process and relational dynamics, interpretation and challenges are often ill-fated, providing little "grist" for the therapeutic mill. Consequently, my challenge as a therapist was to find times and ways in which Mr. Edwards would provide an opportunity to explore his conflicts such that he would not perceive it as a hostile attack.

An interesting dynamic also occurred among Mr. Edwards, my supervisor, and me. Given the emphasis for narcissistic patients on power and authority, there was a strange triangulation, wherein Mr. Edwards was aware of the omniscient eye, so to speak, of the supervisor. This was especially salient shortly after beginning to videotape sessions. Initially, Mr. Edwards was extremely reluctant to allow this, only agreeing after several months of work together and with special clauses written into the consent form, detailing in even more specific terms than were already there, the use of the tape and its destruction. In one of our early taped sessions, I began to notice that Mr. Edwards was, in effect, performing for the camera. His emotions were more blatant, his responses tempered and thought out, and his behavior more nervous. Indeed, he would often glance to the camera and ask if we were taping, especially when exploring a particularly sensitive area. My supervisor and I explored this behavior during our consultations and agreed that it would be valuable to subtly explore the meaning of his change in presentation. The next session, after he exhibited such behaviors, I asked Mr. Edwards if it bothered him that we were taping or if he was worried about the supervisor. He immediately turned to the camera, saying he was not nervous and that he "didn't give a damn what he thought." My supervisor and I found this particularly intriguing, as it seemed to reflect that he *did* worry about situations in which another person may be evaluating him. In this case, the supervisor represented an unknown factor for Mr. Edwards, which made it difficult to determine whether the supervisor was caring, judging, or indifferent. In some ways, it was another projection of his underlying insecurities about being judged by a father-like figure. Further, this episode exemplified the triangulation that is often seen in narcissistic patients. Specifically, Mr. Edwards placed my supervisor and me into a position of tension, wherein his relationship with me (and the special quality of that relationship) was threatened by a powerful third-party that held sway over both him and me. Herein, we see a classic transference wherein I take on a more maternal role, being the individual who is intimate, supportive, communicative, and warm, while the supervisor becomes the father figure, who is less present and available, yet ultimately holds sway over the mother-figure in a more powerful manner than does the patient (i.e., child). Interestingly, this reenacted for Mr. Edwards the reported tensions within his own relationships and development with his parents. Further, Mr. Edwards's reaction pulled for more maternal countertransference behaviors, where I sought to assuage Mr. Edwards's fears or distress about the monitoring by the "father figure." This exchange was valuable, however, in that it allowed

Mr. Edwards and me to candidly discuss how the taping made him feel and whether he was "putting on a show" for the viewer. He admitted he was a bit, but was unable to really articulate why he found it necessary to do so. This would continue to be addressed when needed throughout our work together, especially as it reflected his beliefs about how others perceived him, judged him, and related to him. Nevertheless, this remained until the end of our work together an area of difficulty for Mr. Edwards, who failed to fully develop insight into how he related to others and how he "performed" in an attempt to be accepted by others.

Finally, I noticed at times a strong sense of being paternalistic with Mr. Edwards. His style of interaction—marked by the somewhat unusual behaviors already noted—in combination with the stories he told of how his work and social interactions unfolded—reminded me of the prototypical, office "loner" whom people criticize and use as the punch line of ongoing jokes. Perhaps this was the first indication of countertransference I was developing that made me feel somewhat fatherly or like a caretaker; his depleted-type of narcissism, along with his social awkwardness, odd behaviors, juvenile mentality, and inexperience in life in general, led to a feeling of pity and compassion for him. This reaction also appeared during difficult transitional or developmental periods for Mr. Edwards. For instance, after Mr. Edwards's wife died, I experienced a strong mixed reaction about how he responded to this event. As noted, he initially seemed to be depressed and withdrawn, genuinely mourning her passing; however, within a short period of time, he began speaking explicitly of wanting a new romantic or sexual partner. While I felt a pull to comfort him as a parent would, processing the grief and helping him work through the difficult emotions—again reflecting the underlying parental countertransference, I also felt angry that he could seemingly discard a relationship with such flippancy. This was a time of intense countertransference and attempts, on my part, to aggressively pursue his emotions, focusing him on the reasons for his defenses and what the loss of his wife truly meant. In a sense, my own values—the value of close, monogamous relationships and the importance of addressing intense emotions—combined with a parental countertransference to motivate me to try and guide or teach him.

This was perhaps the most unsettling transference I experienced, as it resulted in me, a therapist in his mid-twenties, becoming the father-figure to a man near forty-years-old. I believe this resulted from my own compassion as well as from a pull from Mr. Edwards for me to become a corrective parental figure, who served as an important self-object, while watching over him and offering some form of narcissistic extension. This countertransference would occasionally cause me to falter in challenges or necessary questioning, to reinforce thoughts or actions that perhaps should be dissuaded, and sometimes threatened to result in becoming entwined too greatly for an effective therapeutic relationship. The struggle to distance myself as the therapist was the toughest, for I wanted to be close to help my patients by comforting them and guiding them to a better life. To manage this countertransference required continued exploration in supervision and through personal reflection outside of session. The ultimate solution was to utilize the compassion I felt for Mr. Edwards as a means of mirroring his own emotions and experiences, helping to form a novel, corrective relationship I spoke to earlier, and to adopt an attitude of curiosity about his experience, his problems, and his growth during our work together.

A final frustration of our therapy was our inability to work toward the natural endpoint of treatment, wherein Mr. Edwards could move beyond dealing with daily struggles and problems toward integration of self-insight concerning his personality and relational dynamics. Mr. Edwards's financial issues, as well as relational functioning, could be addressed to some extent, but the ultimate goal was clearly improved personal insight and ego-functioning. However, this frustration proved to be a sort of blessing, for it brought with it one of my most valuable training lessons. Specifically, throughout our work together, it began to seem that Mr. Edwards's problems were not to be "fixed," but, instead, to be processed to determine the underlying issues that were causing manifest difficulties as well as psychological distress. This was a wonderful lesson for a nervous new therapist: therapy was not simply checking off problems on a list, and providing textbook solutions for common maladies. Instead, therapy was a *dynamic* process, involving an ongoing, evolving communication between the therapist and patient, aimed, hopefully, at resolving the presenting issues, as well as those that may be underlying these complaints. Indeed, McWilliams (1994) noted that there are several important therapist qualities that are necessary when treating narcissistic personalities, including patience, empathy, nonjudgment, realistic evaluation of events, and acknowledgement of our errors and feelings as therapists. Each of these factors was a skill I had to utilize in my treatment with Mr. Edwards, and I value the growth I experienced as a result.

As I grew as a therapist, and as the connection between Mr. Edwards and myself continued to develop, I added to this realization a point that is crucial for all new therapists to recognize: progress is made every session, even when it does not seem so. I was consistently taken aback when Mr. Edwards would come in for a session and it would seem that we made no discernible progress. However, often after these sessions or at the beginning of the following session, Mr. Edwards would comment that he had made a connection or drawn some new insight into a problem. We, as therapists, make a difference in many different ways, one of which is simply *being* with the patient, helping him reflect on and articulate his thoughts, develop new insights and relationships, and actually listen to their stories. Mr. Edwards helped me realize this throughout our treatment together.

SUMMARY

By working with Mr. Edwards, I developed a much stronger sense of my own clinical identity, as well as a deeper understanding of my counter-transferential reactions. I became more confident and comfortable developing relationships with my patients, as well as processing the emotions that develop during the course of therapy and the roles that we enact during our work together.

In addition, the benefits of being open in supervision, acknowledging my emotions and reactions, and processing these with honesty are paramount. My supervisors have been able to explore what I bring to the session, without creating an atmosphere that I feel crosses the boundaries of the supervisory relationship. Balancing disclosure and exploration of self in supervision with the case conceptualization and planning for future therapeutic interactions allows for personal growth as a therapist, as well as gains for the patient. I believe by being honest about my reactions, I was able to shape the therapeutic environment to best help Mr. Edwards move into a corrective relationship, wherein I could begin to explore his past, mirror his emotions and thoughts, and model empathy and reflection. Although progress was sometimes slow, I believe that Mr. Edwards achieved gains in many areas, including intrapersonal insight, as well as gains with his financial problems, while successfully navigating emotional crises like the loss of his wife and his job, confusion about family dynamics, and social alienation. Mr. Edwards improved his ability to approach life with continual optimism and was increasingly willing to explore his identity and the mistakes he had made, as well as identify what progress he had made on successes and personal strengths.

As I write this summary, nearly a year after our mutual termination of treatment, I wonder where Mr. Edwards is, what he is doing, and how he has processed our relationship. I can only hope that our relationship remains internalized as a means by which he will continue to engage in personal development and exploration. Such is the best we can wish of many of our patients, especially when struggling with underlying personality pathology, like narcissism. Likewise, we should as therapists, especially training therapists, utilize these experiences to gain comfort and confidence in working with strong transferential and countertransferential reactions and often-difficult long-term therapy.

NOTES

1. The author would like to acknowledge the following individuals who served as supervisors or consultants in this case: Carol Freedman-Doan, PhD, Norman Gordon, PhD, Nina Nabors, PhD, Karen Saules, PhD, and Michael Shulman, PhD.

2. It should be noted that this does not necessarily equate with the conventions of the current edition of the Diagnostic and Statistical Manual of Mental Disorders's (DSM-IV-TR; American Psychiatric Association (APA), 2000) diagnosis of Narcissistic Personality Disorder (NPD). As noted in Chapter 2, the DSM-IV-TR diagnosis of NPD and the historical conceptualization of narcissism in psychoanalytic theory are markedly different. Psychoanalytic and psychodynamic theory has long held that narcissism, along with other traits, such as hysteria and depression, stem from our developmental experiences and the relations we developed with early caregivers—specifically, the mother-figure (Blatt & Shichman, 1983; Wink, 1991).

REFERENCES

American Psychiatric Association. (2000). *Diagnostic and statistical manual of mental disorders* (4th ed., text revision). Washington, DC: Author.

Blatt, S. J. & Shichman, S. (1983). Two primary configurations of psychopathology. *Psychoanalysis and Contemporary Thought, 6,* 187–254.

Gabbard, G. O. (2000). *Psychodynamic psychiatry,* (3rd ed.). Washington, DC: American Psychiatric Press.

Hotckiss, S. (2005). Key concepts in the theory and treatment of narcissistic phenomena. *Clinical Social Work Journal, 33,* 127–44.

Kernberg, O. (1975). *Borderline conditions and pathological narcissism.* New York, NY: Jason Aronson.

Kernberg, O. (1976). *Object relations theory and clinical psychoanalysis.* New York, NY: Jason Aronson.

Kernberg, O. (1984). *Severe personality disorders: Psychotherapeutic strategies.* New Haven, CT: Yale University Press.

Kohut, H. (1968). The psychoanalytic treatment of narcissistic personality disorders: Outline of a systematic approach. *The Psychoanalytic Study of the Child, 23,* 86–113.

Kohut, H. (1971). *The analysis of the self: A systematic approach to the psychoanalytic treatment of narcissistic personality disorders.* New York, NY: International Universities Press.

Kohut, H. (1977). *The restoration of the self.* New York, NY: International Universities Press.

McWilliams, N. (1994). *Psychoanalytic diagnosis.* New York, NY: Guilford.

Miller, A. (1981). *Prisoners of childhood.* New York, NY: Basic Books.

Schultz, R. E. & Glickauf-Hughes, C. (1995). Countertransference in the treatment of pathological narcissism. *Psychotherapy, 32,* 601–07.

Wink, P. (1991). Two faces of narcissism. *Journal of Personality and Social Psychology, 61*(4), 590–97.

Winnicott, D.W. (1967). Mirror-role of mother and family in child development. In *Playing and reality* (pp. 111–18). New York, NY: Basic Books.

7

Concluding Remarks

Steven K. Huprich

The purpose of this book has been to introduce readers to basic psychodynamic principles of narcissistic pathology, to describe case treatment histories that have targeted narcissistic pathology as a fundamental part of treatment, and to discuss how countertransference feelings and reactions inform treatment in therapeutically productive ways. This has been quite an ambitious undertaking for us all. In the midst of busy semesters, finding time to think, write, and edit this book has been challenging. The project has stretched our collective thinking and understanding of our patients and ourselves. As a result, we feel a deep sense of satisfaction in our accomplishment and hope that our efforts have helped other therapists who work with patients struggling with such conflicts and difficulties. We also feel a deep sense of appreciation to our patients, who courageously have shared their life struggles with us and from whom we have learned much. Their attainment of greater happiness, life satisfaction, and self-understanding is what we all work for, and we trust that their therapeutic examples and gains will help others achieve similar or greater levels gratification.

In reflecting upon what I have observed as a supervisor and consultant in this process, I can say there have been some considerable gains that these authors have experienced in their professional development. These observations have led me to share what I believe to be fundamentals for new therapists who may currently, or eventually will, encounter patients with narcissistic pathology. It is with these fundamentals that I wish to close this chapter.

First, it is very important that new therapists learn about narcissistic pathology and conflicts. The DSM-IV-Text Revision (APA, 2001) and its predecessor have been criticized for failing to capture narcissistic pathology as it has been traditionally understood (Cooper & Michels, 1988; Gunder-son, Ronningstam, & Smith, 1991; McWilliams, 1994). Learning as much as one can about the dynamic and analytic conceptualization of narcissis-tic pathology and personalities provides a much richer and thorough base from which to recognize, understand, and treat narcissistic pathology. Per-sonally, I have found McWilliams' (1994) text to be very helpful to students in this regard.

Second, new therapists benefit tremendously from watching or listening to tapes of their sessions with such patients under the supervision of a sea-soned supervisor. As was demonstrated in the earlier chapters, individuals with narcissistic pathology present themselves in challenging and/or com-plicated ways. Beginning therapists often have trouble recognizing and un-derstanding the content, process, and dynamics commonly observed in these sessions. For instance, what may be understood as a simple and rea-sonable negative reaction to a frustration or disappointment may be a much deeper narcissistic injury or wound that causes much greater conflict and sadness than what may initially present itself. Likewise, the complex patterns of defenses that may raise themselves are often missed.

Related to the above, beginning therapists are very strongly encouraged to be open to sharing their thoughts, feelings, and reactions in the context of clinical supervision. By now it is quite obvious that this text has demon-strated how useful recognizing, identifying, and understanding counter-transference experiences are in working with patients who have narcissistic pathology. It is quite normal and understandable to respond with feelings of shock, disbelief, irritation, boredom, and amusement at the many things one might hear from patients. I think of Ms. Fons's experiences with Mr. Garcia, and his incredibly personal attacks on her appearance early on in treatment, or Mr. Parker's feelings of amusement at the grandiose stories that Mr. Miller's patient told about his daring efforts to rescue and protect others. By knowing one's inner experience of these patients, therapists are in a much better position to understand the function of patients' comments and be more empathic toward the underlying conflict or concern that mo-tivates them.

Fourth, I think it is important for beginning therapists to recognize that, just because patients elicit strong feelings or meet criteria for an Axis II dis-order, this is no reason to back away from treating them or believing they can make meaningful changes in therapy. These new therapists (Ms. Fons, Mr. Brown, Mr. Erdodi, and Mr. Parker) demonstrated courage and re-silience in understanding their patients and finding effective ways of inter-vening with them. Their commitment to their patients and their own edu-cation served them and their patients very well.

Fifth, in this day and age when brief treatments and symptom-focused treatments are emphasized in clinical training programs, there is the unfortunate consequence of dismissing the more complex issues facing patients and addressing these in treatment. Consequently, therapists are less prepared to treat patients with complex and difficult problems (such as these) and sadly relegate their problems to the pejorative position of being "characterological" without the recognition that such problems can be effectively treated and understood. Yet, as has been well documented in the literature (Westen & Novotny, & Thompson-Brenner, 2004), most patients do not come to therapy with one focal problem that is relatively well contained in its effect on their lives. Most have a set of problems that are interrelated and a product of well-established personality patterns. As was seen in Mr. Edwards's and Mr. Garcia's cases, interventions that were based upon empirically supported interventions did not provide meaningful results. In fact, they produced a rift in the therapeutic relationship and patients' beliefs that therapy could be helpful. Fortunately, longer-term, empirically supported interventions are being reported for patients with personality disorders (Huprich, 2008; Leichsenring, 2006; Levy et al., 2006; Porcerelli, Dauphin, Ablon, Leitman, & Bambery, 2007; Sandell, Blomberg, Lazar, Carlsson, Broberg, & Schubert, 2000) and problems with the assumptions behind most of the empirically supported movement are being recognized (Morrison, Bradley, & Westen, 2003; Westen, et al., 2004). Therefore, it is important for new therapists to be very cognizant of the fact that long-term treatment of personality pathology is effective and a necessary component of their training.

Fifth, and related to the above, meaningful change can and does occur with patients who have narcissistic pathology. For instance, these cases have demonstrated that patients can and do experience an effective decrease and remission of suicidal ideation, self-destructive tendencies, and physical and verbal aggression. They also were able to develop a more coherent sense of self that acts out of reason and choice instead of being shaped by the world and experiences around them. They also were able to more effectively cope with the death of loved ones compared to when they began treatment.

Finally, as the authors themselves have articulated, therapists learn a tremendous amount about themselves as persons. For instance, it comes as a surprise to many new therapists that, having considered themselves to be kind and caring individuals, they have feelings of dislike, irritation, or frustration with a patient. This knowledge directly contradicts what almost all new therapists have believed about themselves; yet, this knowledge does not mean that they cannot be effective or that they cannot overcome these initial feelings. Rather, it validates and enriches their understanding of themselves as human beings with a rich, inner life which dynamically interacts with the world around them. It expands their sense of what it means to be human and that ambivalent feelings need not be viewed as problematic, but as something to be understood and appreciated.

Most new therapists also learn that their pre-conceived ideas about what therapy is must be changed in order to fit their experiences of what works with patients who have narcissistic pathology. Incongruence between the therapy room experience and one's inner representation of psychotherapy is quite typical, and often hard for new therapists to fully recognize and accept. Too often, new therapists wish to hang on tenaciously to what they have read and been told about therapy; yet, time and time again, what the patient brings to the therapy room fails to fit nicely into that representation. For example, many of my supervisees tell me that they do not believe therapy is going well because "nothing that significant happened" in treatment, which means that the patient did not talk about things that lent themselves readily to some form of intervention that targeted key areas that maintained their psychopathology, such as their impaired object relations or core schemas. All too often, this elicits distress and anxiety in new therapists, with the belief that there is something deficient and inadequate inside of them—that they must be doing something wrong or not working hard enough. Yet, this incongruence does not need to be viewed as a narcissistic threat to one's skills or professional integrity. Rather, it can be understood as an opportunity to learn and develop within a supportive and caring supervisory relationship. In other words, new therapists must learn how to work through their own narcissistic challenges in order to be effective with their narcissistic patients. Thus, part of the work of learning to work with narcissistic patients is learning to work through one's own narcissistic threats to one's sense of esteem and agency. Without this, therapists are likely to feel frustrated by their patients' resistance and defenses, as well as what all these elicit.

In conclusion, it is my sincere hope that this text book has been helpful for new or seasoned therapists who find working with narcissistic patients to be challenging. By recognizing and understanding narcissistic pathology and the reactions it elicits, therapists can become more equipped to tolerate, understand, and intervene with patients who usually are viewed as quite challenging and frustrating. Meaningful therapeutic change can and does occur when therapists get comfortable with themselves in the context of their relationship with their patients. Just as narcissistic patients have trouble living with themselves, so do new therapists who are being asked to treat them. Getting more comfortable with one's inner life and understanding it fosters personal and professional growth and makes one a better therapist. What more could one want?

REFERENCES

American Psychiatric Association (2001). *Diagnostic and statistical manual of mental disorders* (4th ed. Text Revision). Washington, DC: Author.

Cooper, A. M., & Michels, R. (1988). Book review of Diagnostic and Statistical Manual of Mental Disorders, 3rd edition, Revised (DSM-III-R by the American Psychiatric Association. *American Journal of Psychiatry, 145,* 1300–01.

Gunderson, J., Ronningstam, E., & Smith, L. (1991). Narcissistic personality disorder: A review of data on DSM-III descriptions. *Journal of Personality Disorders, 5,* 167–77.

Huprich, S. K. (2008, in press). *Psychodynamic therapy: Conceptual and empirical foundations.* New York: Taylor and Francis.

Leichsenring, F. (2006). Review of meta-analyses of outcome studies of psychodynamic therapy. In PDM Task Force, *Psychodynamic diagnostic manual* (pp. 819–37). Silver Spring, MD: Alliance of Psychoanalytic Organizations.

Levy, K. N., Meehan, K. B., Kelly, K. M., Reynoso, J. S., Weber, M. Clarkin, J., et al. (2006). Change in attachment patterns and reflective functioning in a randomized control trial of transference-focused psychotherapy for borderline personality disorder. *Journal of Consulting and Clinical Psychology, 74,* 1027–40.

McWilliams, N. (1994). *Psychoanalytic diagnosis.* New York: Guilford.

Milrod, B., Leon, A. C., Busch, F., Rudden, M., Schwalberg, M., Clarkin, J., et al. (2007). A randomized controlled clinical trail of psychoanalytic psychotherapy for panic disorder. *American Journal of Psychiatry, 164,* 265–72.

Morrison, C., Bradley, R., & Westen, D. (2003). The external validity of efficacy trials for depression and anxiety: A naturalistic study. *Psychology and Psychotherapy: Theory, Research, and Practice, 76,* 109–32.

Porcerelli, J. H., Dauphin, V. B., Ablon, J. S., Leitman, S., & Bambery, M. (2007). Psychoanalysis with avoidant personality disorder: A systematic case study. *Psychotherapy: Theory / Research / Practice / Training, 44,* 1–13.

Sandell, R., Blomberg, J., Lazar, A., Carlsson, J., Broberg, J., & Schubert, J. (2000). Varieties of long-term outcome among patients in psychoanalysis and long-term psychotherapy: A review of findings in the Stockholm Outcome of Psychoanalysis and Psychotherapy Project (STOPP). *International Journal of Psychoanalysis, 81,* 921–42.

Westen, D., Novotny, C. M., & Thompson-Brenner, H. (2004). The empirical status of empirically supported psychotherapies: Assumptions, findings, and reporting in controlled clinical trials. *Psychological Bulletin, 130,* 633–63.

Index

abandonment, fears of, 24, 25, 36–37
absence, parental, 74
abuse of animals, 76–77
academic achievement, 28, 77–78
acceptance, of self, 12, 37, 92
advice for new therapists, 44, 119,
    123–26
affects: Mr. Garcia, 33; Mr. Miller, 52,
    54, 60; Mr. Schultz, 84–85
affirmation, external, 11, 25, 63–64, 98
aggression, displaced, 76–77. *See also*
    violence, of patients
Akhtar, S., 72
alliance. *See* therapeutic alliance
ambiguity: discomfort with, 36, 48; in
    therapy, 36, 43, 89, 107
amusement reaction, 63, 64, 65, 124
anecdotes. *See* storytelling/exaggeration
anger issues, 48, 54, 55
autoeroticism, 5, 6
Axis I and II conditions, 71, 75, 87, 90,
    91

benefits of narcissism, 10
"black/white" thinking. *See* splitting
body language, 30, 39, 40
borderline personality disorder,
    comparisons, 7

boredom: patients', 59–60, 72, 78;
    therapists', in treatment, 16, 41,
    64–65, 109, 114–15
boundary issues: Mr. Edwards, 96,
    118–19; Mr. Schultz, 70–71, 84
bullying, perceived, 108, 109

Carroll, L., 12
cases: Mr. Edwards, 95–122; Mr. Garcia,
    23–46; Mr. Miller, 47–68; Mr.
    Schultz, 69–94
challenging. *See* confrontation, as
    therapy component
change of therapists, 25, 29, 70, 82,
    112
character organization, 7, 55
character pathology, 48, 54
child abuse, 26, 27, 73, 74, 76; effects,
    33–34
child development, 8–9, 14–15, 16–17,
    98; defenses during, 109; discipline,
    33–34
child/parent relationships, 7, 8, 9,
    14–15, 15–18; lack of parental
    empathy/attention, 72–73, 98; Mr.
    Edwards as son, 96–97, 98, 101–2;
    Mr. Garcia as father, 24, 25, 32–34,
    36; Mr. Garcia as son, 26–27,

31–33, 35; Mr. Miller as son, 49–50, 51; Mr. Schultz as son, 70, 73, 74–77; therapeutic relationship as, 19, 62, 64. *See also* father; father figures; mother; mother figures

clinical presentation. *See* presentation

clinical training. *See* training

clinicians. *See* therapists

completion of therapy, 73, 93, 112, 119. *See also* outcomes of treatment

conceptualization, 3, 99–100, 124; challenges, 69; Mr. Edwards, 98, 106, 107, 114, 116; Mr. Schultz, 71–72, 78, 87; of transference, 16–17

confidence levels, therapist, 42, 89, 91, 97, 114, 120

confrontation: in Kernbergian theory, 20, 99, 116; as therapy component, 16, 19, 72, 73, 85, 112, 116–17

confrontation/empathy treatment debate, 73, 99, 116

control issues: defenses for maintaining control, 75, 90; of emotions, 36, 48, 51, 53, 57–58, 89; parents and children, 34, 36; patients and therapists, 15, 39, 42, 70–71, 84; self-control, 12, 49–50; sexual, 34–35, 56

conversations, narcissists', 13, 42. *See also* interpersonal relationships; storytelling/exaggeration

countertransference, 14–18; defined, 87–88; interfering with performance, 89; as learning tool, 88–91, 113; Mr. Edwards case, 113–19; Mr. Garcia case, 38–44; Mr. Miller case, 63–66; Mr. Schultz case, 87–91. *See also* transference

covert narcissism, 12, 13–14, 47; Mr. Schultz, 73, 84

creativity, 79

criteria. *See* DSM-IV

criticism, narcissists' reactions to, 13; Mr. Edwards, 103; Mr. Garcia, 25, 26, 30, 37; Mr. Miller, 62; Mr. Schultz, 76–77, 80, 86

death: family, 51, 58, 61, 62, 75, 102, 109–11; fear of, 60

debt, 95, 106

defenses, 7; grandiosity as, 13; mechanisms, 37, 50–51, 75, 99, 107, 108–9, 115–16; responses to, 19. *See also* specific defenses

demographics of patients, 11

denial: defense, 48, 99, 102, 108, 115; of transference, 15

depleted narcissism, 96, 98, 100, 114

depression: addressed in therapy, 52, 54, 60, 83; as reason for entering therapy, 10–11, 23, 47

devalued narcissism. *See* depleted narcissism

devaluing: addressing, in treatment, 19; by Mr. Garcia, 29–30, 31; by Mr. Schultz, 81; of relationships, 10; of therapists, generally, 15–16, 19–20

developmental arrest, 18, 72

Diagnostic and Statistical Manual of Mental Disorder. *See* DSM-IV

dichotomous thinking, 101. *See also* splitting

"difficult to treat" patients, 2, 38, 69

dominance/submission, sexual, 34–35, 56

drama. *See* melodrama exploitation

DSM-IV: criteria unmet, 71, 100; criticisms of, 123–24; narcissism disorder criteria, 11, 12, 22, 121n2; pathological gambling definition, 106

duality, demonstrated in patients, 74, 83, 84–85

duration of therapy. *See* timeframes for therapy

dynamic perspective/theory, 97, 98–99; therapy based on, 107–8, 116

Eagle, M. N., 87–88

Echo (character), 5

educational backgrounds, patients, 28, 77–78

Edwards, Mr.: background information, 101–4; case description, 95–97; countertransference with, 113–19;

theoretical foundations, 98–101; treatment history, 105–13

ego, 5, 99, 113; structure formation, 18; undeveloped, 48

Ellis, H., 5

emotions: avoidance of, 47–48, 50, 53, 54, 57–59; control, 36, 51, 57–58, 89; explanation/education, 54–55, 59; lack of familial demonstration, 50, 74, 76, 77; management goal, 73, 92; therapists', 87, 113

empathy: demonstrated by patients, 37; demonstrated for patients, 20, 30–31, 38, 41, 42–43, 89–90, 91, 100, 118; lacking in parents (theory), 72–73; lacking in patients, 11, 48, 61; vs. confrontation, in treatment, 73, 99, 116

employment challenges: Mr. Edwards, 95–96, 111; Mr. Schultz, 71, 79, 80, 85

ethnicity, 28, 30, 31

exhibitionism, 34–35

experience, therapists. *See* inexperience and insecurity

extensions, narcissistic, 72–73, 78, 82–83, 98, 103, 118

family relations. *See* child/parent relationships; father; mother; siblings

fantasies: Mr. Edwards, 103–8; Mr. Garcia, 27, 35, 36; Mr. Miller, 47, 48, 51; Mr. Schultz, 85; therapists, 39–40, 42

fathers: of Mr. Edwards, 96–97, 104; of Mr. Garcia, 35–36; of Mr. Miller, 50, 51; of Mr. Schultz, 74, 75, 77; father figures: Mr. Edwards, 106–7, 108, 116, 117, 118; Mr. Schultz, 80

fear of success, 77, 78

feedback, positive, 72, 78

feelings. *See* emotions

financial problems, 95, 96, 105–6, 111, 113–14

free will, 57

Freud, Sigmund: ideas and influence, 5–6, 8–9; on transference, 14, 15

frustrations, of treating narcissistic patients, 15–16, 38–39, 109, 114–15, 116

Gabbard, G. O., 13, 71, 99

gambling addiction, 106

Garcia, Mr.: background, 26–29; case description, 23–26; countertransference with, 38–44; treatment history, 29–37

gender: and diagnosis, 11–12; and patient-therapist relationships, 29, 30, 34, 69

glamour by association, 82–83

Glickauf-Hughes, C., 113, 115

Grandiose-Exhibitionist narcissism, 83. *See also* overt narcissism

grandiose narcissism, 98

grandiosity: Mr. Edwards, 107–8, 110; Mr. Garcia, 25, 37; Mr. Miller, 47, 48, 52, 53; Mr. Schultz, 72, 78, 83–84; and self-esteem, 8; varying levels, 9–10, 12

grieving: Mr. Edwards, 110–11, 118; Mr. Miller, 51, 58, 62

help from supervisors, on countertransference, 124; Mr. Edwards, 115; Mr. Garcia, 40, 42, 43; Mr. Miller, 65; Mr. Schultz, 88, 90–91

"hero" identity fantasy, 47, 50, 51, 52, 55, 59, 62–63

history, narcissistic personality disorder, 5–6

Hotchkiss, S., 98, 99, 109

id, 48, 113

idealization: idealized object, 13; of parents, 16–18, 26–27; and self-image, 7, 16; of therapists, 19, 106, 108, 109, 116

identification with patient, 89–90, 91

inexperience and insecurity, 42–43, 88, 90, 91, 114, 126

inferiority feelings, 11, 13, 84, 100

intellectualization, as defense, 53, 58–59, 65–66, 71

internalization: of grandiosity, 8;
    transmuting, 8, 17, 19
interpersonal relationships: challenged,
    via narcissism, 11, 13; Mr. Edwards,
    103; Mr. Garcia, 28, 37, 41–42; Mr.
    Miller, 55, 58; Mr. Schultz, 74–75,
    82–83; quality evaluation, 10. *See
    also* romantic relationships; social
    impairment (Mr. Edwards); work
    relationships
intuition, therapist, 87
investigations and trials, 5–6, 12

Jacobs, T. J., 88
jealousy: parental, 75–76, 77; of
    patients, 101, 102, 104

Kernberg, Otto: on character pathology,
    48, 98–99; theories, 6–7, 9, 14–15,
    72; on treatment, 16, 19–20. *See also*
    confrontation/empathy treatment
    debate
Klonsky, E. D., 11
Kohut, Heinz: theories, 7, 8, 9, 72–73,
    98–99; on transference, 16–17; on
    treatment, 18–19, 73, 87; on values,
    59. *See also* confrontation/empathy
    treatment debate

libidinal energy, 6
literature: anonymous patient
    depiction, 97; influential, 5–7, 41;
    recommended specific, 124. *See also*
    specific authors
loneliness, 76
long-term therapy, 87, 112, 124–25.
    See also timeframes for therapy
love, capacity, 99

manipulation: by patients, 105, 108; of
    patients, 48, 57, 65, 104
marriage: Mr. Garcia, 24, 27; of parents,
    75, 76. *See also* spouses
masculinity, 35, 56, 63, 95, 104, 111
McWilliams, Nancy, 15, 41, 72, 98,
    113, 114–15
medical ailments: Mr. Garcia, 24–25,
    28–29; Mr. Miller, 49

melodrama exploitation, 51, 55, 58,
    59–60
mental illness, family, 75, 77
Metamorphoses (Ovid), 5
Miller, Mr.: background and treatment,
    49–52; case description, 47–48;
    countertransference with, 63–66;
    treatment history, 52–63
Minnesota Multiphasic Personality
    Disorder (MMPD) scales, 12
Minnesota Multiphasic Personality
    Inventory (MMPI), 100
mirroring, 8, 16–18, 116; usage, 19, 31,
    54, 98
mirror transference, 115
monitoring, visual, of therapists, 40,
    41, 65, 116, 117–18; utilization in
    education, 124
mothers: of Mr. Edwards, 101; Mr.
    Garcia, 26–27; Mr. Miller, 49–50,
    51–52; Mr. Schultz, 75–76
mother figures, 102–3, 104, 110
motivation of patients, 2–3, 70, 84,
    109; lacking, 43, 73

narcissistic personality disorder: clinical
    presentation, 10–12; defined/traits,
    72, 73, 83–84, 99; diagnostic
    criteria, 11, 12, 22, 121n2; forms,
    12–14, 83, 98–99; history, 5–6;
    normative vs. pathological, 9–10;
    theories, 6–9; treatment, 18–20
narcissists: defined/described, 7, 11, 72,
    98; described by Kernberg, 7, 99;
    described by Kohut, 99; McWilliams
    on, 99–100
Narcissus (character), 5
narratives of patients, 70, 77, 78, 82,
    86. *See also* storytelling/exaggeration
Nemesis (character), 5
normal/pathological disorder, 9–10
NPD. *See* narcissistic personality
    disorder

objectification of patients, 97
object love, 6, 9
object relations, 8–9; development, 15,
    19; theory, 98

Oltmanns, T. E., 11
On Narcissism (Freud), 5–6
outcomes of treatment, 19, 125; Mr.
  Edwards, 112–13, 120; Mr. Garcia,
  37; Mr. Miller, 61–63, 66–67; Mr.
  Schultz, 86–87, 92
overt narcissism, 12, 13–14, 47; Mr.
  Schultz, 73, 83–85
Ovid, 5

parent/child relationships. *See*
  child/parent relationships
parent imago, 18
parents of narcissists. *See* child/parent
  relationships
pathological/normal disorder, 9–10
Personality Disorder NOS, 71
pessimism, on treating narcissism, 6
power dynamic, patient/therapist, 39, 42,
  63, 70–71. *See also* boundary issues
presentation: clinical, 10–12; Mr.
  Edwards, 95, 100, 117; Mr. Garcia,
  24; Mr. Miller, 52; Mr. Schultz, 69,
  73, 81, 83–85, 92
prestige, of relationships, 82–83
primary narcissism, 6, 9
process variables, 114, 115
professionalism, perceived, 23, 38, 39,
  126. *See also* confidence levels,
  therapist
progress of therapy: Mr. Edwards, 106,
  112, 119; Mr. Miller, 52, 62, 65; Mr.
  Schultz, 73–74, 81–82, 86, 91
projection examples, 19, 31, 33, 34, 117
pseudovitality, 73
psychic structures, 13, 18, 19
psychoanalytic theory, 4n1, 121n2
psychodynamic theory, 3, 4n1, 121n2

qualities needed, in therapists, 119

racial issues, 28
Racker, H., 14, 20n1, 88
rage, 15, 19, 91
reaction monitoring. *See* monitoring,
  visual, of therapists
reasons for entering therapy, 10–11, 23,
  47, 69, 95

recorded sessions, reviewing, 40, 41, 65
Reich, A., 6, 9–10, 12
relationships. *See* child/parent
  relationships; interpersonal
  relationships; romantic
  relationships; work relationships
religious beliefs, influence, 24, 27
repetition, of stories, 86, 96, 100, 115
rescue fantasies, 39–40, 42
resistance, transference as, 14–16
romantic relationships: Mr. Edwards,
  103–4; Mr. Garcia, 24, 27; Mr.
  Schultz, 71, 79–80, 81
Rose, P., 13

sadism and masochism, 34–35, 56
schizophrenia, 9
Schultz, Mr.: background information,
  74–81; case description, 69–74;
  countertransference with, 87–91;
  treatment history, 81–87
Schultz, R. E., 113, 115
secondary narcissism, 6
secondary outcomes of disorder, 9–10
self-acceptance, 12, 37, 92
self-doubt, 70, 74, 81, 85
self-efficacy, 61, 62, 105
self-esteem: and grandiosity, 8, 13, 37;
  maintenance, 13–14, 81, 85; of
  therapists, 40–41; of young people,
  16–17, 96
self-image, 7, 57, 60, 72, 78, 85
self-narratives. *See* narratives of patients
self-objects, 9, 99; spouses as, 103, 110;
  therapists as, 16, 18, 106, 115, 116
self-referrals, 69
sense of self, 3–4; development, 8,
  16–17; in narcissists, 7, 9–10, 40,
  59; repairing, 19, 113
sexual issues: avoidance of discussion,
  55–56; control-related, 34–35, 56;
  frustration, 95; orientation, 23, 24,
  27, 102; preoccupation/
  inappropriateness, 96, 102, 103–4,
  110–11
shame feelings, 70, 76, 96, 99
siblings: Mr. Edwards, 98, 101–2; Mr.
  Schultz, 74, 77

social impairment (Mr. Edwards), 95,
96, 100–101, 110–11, 118
split representations. *See* duality,
demonstrated in patients
splitting defense, 35, 48, 54, 99, 108
spouses: Mr. Edwards, 98, 102–3, 104,
109–10; Mr. Garcia, 24; ratings by, 12
stepparents, 76
storytelling/exaggeration: Mr. Edwards,
96, 100, 115; Mr. Garcia, 25, 31; Mr.
Miller, 47, 51, 63, 65; Mr. Schultz,
71, 78, 84
structural deficit, 73
submission/dominance, sexual, 34–35,
36
subtypes of narcissism, 83–84, 98–99
suicide: attempts, 47, 60; of family, 77;
ideation, 23, 28, 31–32, 52
superego: deficits in functioning, 99;
developing, 18; therapist as, 113;
undeveloped, 48
supervision: countertransference advice,
38, 40, 42, 43, 65, 88, 90–91, 115;
first-person accounts, 1, 3, 123–26;
group, 41, 116; patient awareness
of, 117

taping. *See* monitoring, visual, of
therapists
therapeutic alliance, 14, 15;
establishing, 90, 95, 100; Mr. Garcia,
29–31, 42, 43; Mr. Miller, 61; Mr.
Schultz, 71, 73, 82, 86, 92–93
therapists: additional benefits for, 4,
125; changing, 25, 29, 70, 82, 112;
inexperience/insecurity, 42–43, 88,
90, 91, 114, 126; Mr. Garcia's
reactions to, 23–24, 25, 29–31, 34,
36, 37, 39, 42; Mr. Miller's reactions
to, 61–62; Mr. Schultz's reactions
to, 86, 88, 90; narcissistic
challenges within, 18, 126; patients'
reactions to, 14, 15–16, 18;
qualities for successful, 119;
training, 2, 3, 4n1, 38, 112; values,
in practice, 40–41. *See also*
confrontation, as therapy

component; countertransference;
empathy; training
Thomson, J. A., 72
Three Essays on the Theory of Sexuality
(Freud), 5
timeframes for therapy, 81–82, 87, 97
tragic hero role. *See* "hero" identity
fantasy
training, 2, 3, 4n1, 38, 112
transference, 14–18; mirror, 115;
patients' denials, 15; sexualized, 34.
See also countertransference;
devaluing; idealization
transfers. *See* change of therapists
transmuting internalization, 8, 17, 19
trauma experiences: Mr. Miller, 55; Mr.
Schultz, 70, 74, 75, 76;
recounting/discussing, 82, 86
treatment, narcissistic personality
disorder, 18–20; feasibility, 6;
outcomes, 19, 92, 125. *See also*
confrontation/empathy treatment
debate; specific cases
Turkheimer, E., 11
types of therapy, 69, 105

underemployment, 80, 83
understanding. *See* empathy
U-tube analogy (Freud), 6

values: mesh of patient's and
therapist's, 40–41; patients'
internal/external, 59
variables, process-related, 114, 115
victimization examples: Mr. Garcia, 31;
Mr. Miller, 50, 56–57
violence, of patients, 47, 50, 51, 76–77
Vulnerable-Sensitive narcissism, 83. *See
also* covert narcissism

weaknesses: concealing, 57; emotions
as, 51, 57, 62; exposed by others, 76
Wink, P., 12, 72, 83, 98
Winnicott, D. W., 59
work relationships: Mr. Edwards, 95–96,
111; Mr. Garcia, 24, 25, 28, 31, 36.
See also employment challenges
writings, influential, 5–7, 41